THE CSIRO
HEALTHY GUT DIET

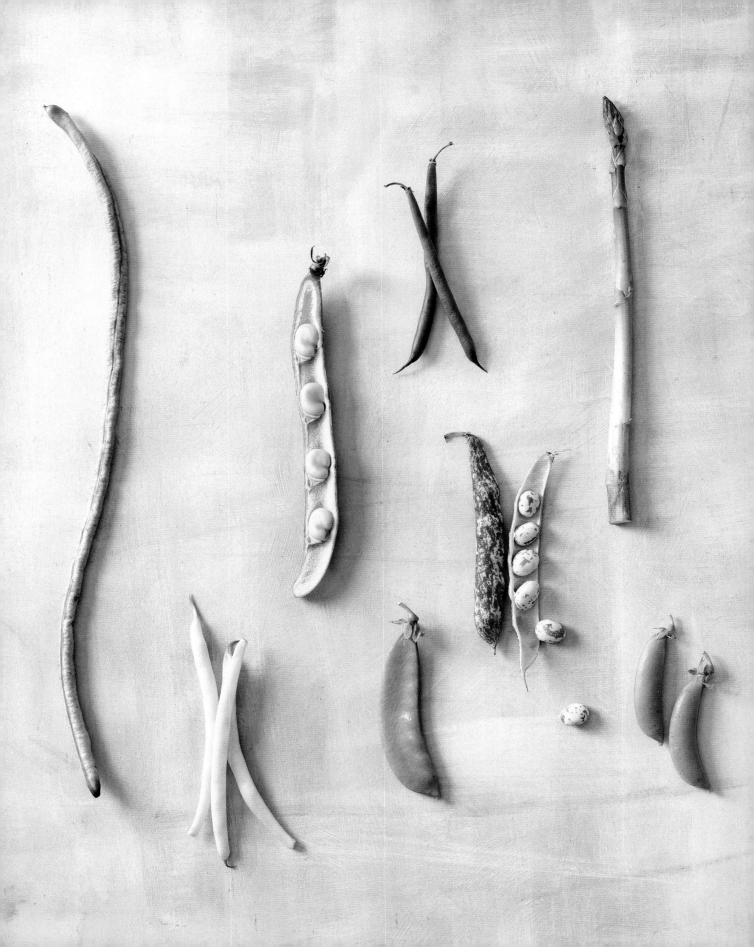

THE CSIRO HEALTHY GUT DIET

Dr Tony Bird, Dr Michael Conlon and Pennie Taylor

Photography by
Rob Palmer

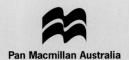

Pan Macmillan Australia

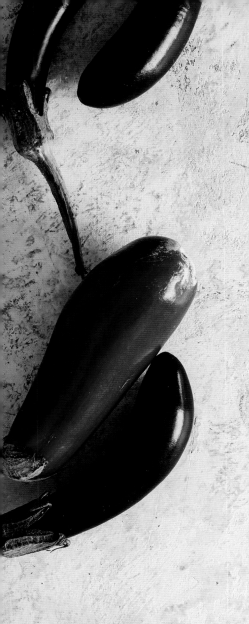

contents

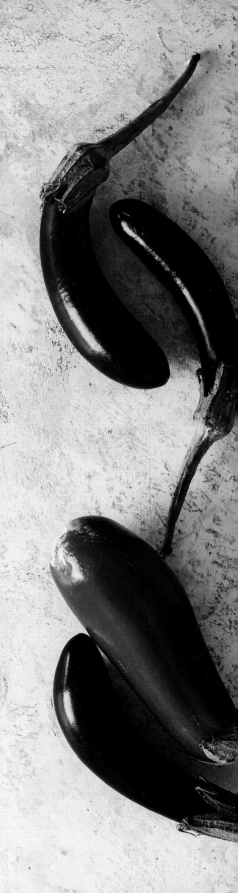

About *the* authors

Dr Tony Bird

Tony is a Principal Research Scientist at CSIRO Health and Biosecurity where he leads multidisciplinary research teams investigating the influences of foods and food constituents on human health and wellbeing, with particular emphasis on dietary fibre and its role in reducing chronic disease risk.

He has more than 35 years' of research experience and his recent activities have centred on advancing the understanding of the nutritional properties and health benefits of cereal foods and grain constituents, their influence on gut microbiota composition and metabolic activity, and their role in regulating the physiology, endocrinology and function of the gastrointestinal tract. For most of that time he has worked extensively with food companies and academia to translate research findings into improved products and practices for promoting population nutrition and health.

Tony is the author of more than 200 scientific articles, reviews and book chapters, and is recognised nationally and internationally for his contribution to the area of dietary fibre and human health research. His awards include the CSIRO Medal for Research Achievement and the Kenneth R. Keller Award for Excellence in Graduate Research. He currently serves as a member of the Scientific Advisory Committee of *The Lancet Gastroenterology & Hepatology*.

Dr Michael Conlon

Michael is a Senior Research Scientist at CSIRO Health and Biosecurity, with a PhD in biochemistry from the University of Adelaide. He has more than 30 years' experience in conducting pre-clinical and clinical research studies, many of which relate to diet and health.

A focus of his work has been on understanding the effects of dietary components such as fibres and proteins on gut physiology (and ultimately other tissues and systems of the body) through their influence on the growth and activities of large bowel microbes. He has been instrumental in conducting a series of studies which have shown that inclusion of resistant starch in the diet can help protect against a toxic environment and tissue damage within the large bowel induced through poor diets common in Western societies. These studies have also shown the importance of gut fermentation in producing the short-chain fatty acids which help maintain large bowel health. He has also carried out numerous studies involving probiotics and prebiotics. This research has been applied to understanding and helping prevent conditions such as inflammatory bowel disease and colorectal cancer.

Pennie Taylor

Pennie is a Research Dietitian/Scientist in the Nutrition and Health program at CSIRO Health and Biosecurity. She completed her PhD in 2018 at the University of Adelaide School of Medicine and also holds a Master's degree in nutrition and dietetics at Flinders University. Pennie's experience spans diet design for complex clinical trials to the development of community weight management and chronic disease programs, specialising in obesity, diabetes, cardiovascular diseases and weight-loss surgery. She translates research outcomes into nutrition and health strategies for relevant segments in the community, and is the co-author of *The CSIRO Low-Carb Diet* and *CSIRO Low Carb Every Day*.

Working with industry partners to adapt science into clinical and community outcomes, her interest is in strategies to optimise glucose control, appetite response and eating behaviours. Pennie is recognised nationally for her contribution to the Dietitians Association Australia's bariatric nutrition program development and as a member of the Australian and New Zealand Metabolic and Obesity Surgery Society.

About *the* contributors

Dr David Topping

David is a post-retirement Fellow at CSIRO Health and Biosecurity. He has more than 40 years' research experience in investigating the relationship between dietary fibre and gastrointestinal function. He has pioneered the concept that many of the beneficial actions of fibre components are effected through the products of their fermentation by the large bowel microbiome and that current intakes of fermentable fibre components are low. As well as investigating the beneficial actions of these products, the short-chain fatty acids, he has worked with CSIRO and academic colleagues and food industry to increase the range of consumer foods containing fermentable fibres.

David is the author of more than 190 scientific papers, reviews and book chapters and 11 patent disclosures, including the invention of high amylose barley and wheat, both of which are undergoing commercial development internationally. He is a deputy editor of the *British Journal of Nutrition* and a reviewer for several other journals and also for national and international granting agencies. He has been recognised by honorary membership of the Grains for Health Foundation in the United States and three CSIRO Medals for Research and Commercialisation Achievement. He is a Past President and a Fellow of the Nutrition Society of Australia and a Fellow of the Academy of Science and Engineering.

Dr Trevor Lockett

Trevor is Managing Director and CEO of biotech company Rhythm Biosciences Limited which develops new diagnostic tests for bowel cancer. A molecular biologist by training, Trevor received his PhD in biochemistry from the University of Adelaide and postdoctoral experience at the Rockefeller University in New York. He has over 30 years' diverse research experience, predominantly at the CSIRO, where he led large multidisciplinary research efforts in the areas of prostate cancer gene therapy, colorectal cancer prevention and the promotion of gastro-intestinal health. In his roles as Theme Leader, Colorectal Cancer and Gut Health, and Group Leader for Personalised Health, Trevor oversaw the research efforts of teams developing new diagnostic tests for the early detection of bowel cancer and investigating the interaction between foods and dietary components, particularly dietary fibre, and human health, including via their impact on the gut microbiome.

During his time at the CSIRO Trevor published in excess of 90 peer-reviewed scientific papers and book chapters, was an inventor of seven active patent families (all of which were licensed), and served on the leadership executive team of a number of business units within the CSIRO. Trevor has a strong commitment to improving human health and wellbeing through the translation and commercialisation of scientific discovery into innovative products and services.

Dr Julie Clarke

Julie is a Senior Research Scientist in the Nutritional Interventions program at CSIRO Health and Biosecurity. She has over 30 years' experience in biomedical research focusing on aspects of gastrointestinal health.

Julie's role for the past 15 years has included Project Leader for CSIRO's acylated starch technology. Acylated starches deliver short chain fatty acids (SCFA) to the large bowel and Julie and her team have focused on the effects of SCFA on gut function and disease prevention and treatment. She is Project Leader for the multi-state, complex clinical trial. Other key clinical studies Julie has been involved with include the effects of the acylated starches on acute infectious diarrhoea, irritable bowel syndrome, immune function of athletes, ulcerative colitis and induction of long-term tolerance in peanut-allergic children. She has attracted over $3.7 million in grants to support her research.

Julie's research with her Japanese and Monash collaborators has advanced our understanding of the influence of the gut microbiota and diet on allergic and inflammatory disease resulting in three publications in *Nature*. She is recognised internationally as a lead scientist in the field of health effects of short chain fatty acids and their clinical potential.

Megan Rebuli

Megan is an experienced Research Dietitian in the Nutrition Interventions team at CSIRO Health and Biosecurity. Megan has a background in public health nutrition and epidemiology, as well as extensive knowledge in dietary assessment and treatment in practice. Megan is involved in a number of clinical trials including weight loss, cardiovascular disease, diabetes, and general nutrition. Her interests lie in chronic disease prevention, dietary patterns and influencing behavior change to improve health outcomes.

Her current role includes analysing dietary data including clinical trials and population survey data; delivery and evaluation of community and public health nutrition interventions and initiatives and literature reviews for health claim substantiations. She was a contributor to *The CSIRO Low-Carb Diet*, and has worked on the development, validation and ongoing evaluation of the CSIRO diet score.

Dr Domenico Sergi

Domenico is a Postdoctoral Research Fellow at CSIRO Health and Biosecurity. He completed his PhD in human nutrition at the Rowett Institute of Nutrition and Health (Scotland, UK) and holds a Bachelor as well as a Master's degree in science of nutrition.

Domenico's expertise is in molecular biology and nutrition with a genuine interest in the effect of nutrients and other food components on metabolic health, energy metabolism and the regulation of energy balance. He is particularly interested in the role of lipotoxicity in metabolic health. His main interest lies in the mechanisms underpinning the development of obesity and its comorbidities. He is passionate about understanding the modulation of key patho-physiological pathways which have been proved to be deleterious for metabolic health.

Domenico has co-authored a book chapter on the effect of nutrition on the brain and presented his research findings at international conferences and meetings held in Scotland, China and New Zealand.

Dr Cuong D Tran

Cuong is a Senior Research Scientist at CSIRO Health and Biosecurity, and an Affiliate Senior Lecturer at the University of Adelaide. He has a PhD in nutritional physiology and gastroenterology, and over 15 years' research experience in nutrition, gut disorders and health. Cuong has a particular interest in developing effective diagnostic measures of gut health and function, such as the gut barrier test, and how that impacts on health and wellbeing. He has published almost 50 peer-reviewed research papers on the topic of zinc nutrition as a potential therapy for inflamed conditions of the gut, non-invasive testing for gut health, and small bowel integrity and function.

Cuong is currently working on commercialising his gut health test to improve public health through an ON Accelerator Program powered by CSIRO, which will be made available to the public. For further information on the team and the diagnostic test please visit us at research.csiro.au/guthealthco/

Dr Damien Belobrajdic

Damien is a Senior Research Scientist at CSIRO Health and Biosecurity. He has a PhD in physiology, and more than 15 years' experience conducting pre-clinical and clinical nutritional trials. He looks at how food and food ingredients can reduce our risk of metabolic disease by improving gut health. In the last decade, his research has focused on substantiating the metabolic health benefits of novel cereal grains and their component carbohydrates, and in providing a deeper understanding of the mechanisms of their benefit. A core focus of this work has been to deliver premium grain and grain-based foods that provide significant socioeconomic benefits for Australia.

Damien has authored over 30 peer-reviewed articles, a book chapter, numerous industry reports and a patent. He has received awards from the International Association for Cereal Science and Technology, the Australian Academy of Science, the Australian Society of Medical Research and the Nutrition Society of Australia. He currently serves on the management committees of the Oceanic Nutrition Leaders Platform and the Complaints Advisory Committee for the Grains and Legumes Nutrition Council.

Dr Sinead Golley

Sinead is a behavioural scientist who joined the CSIRO in May 2009. Her particular expertise lies in the areas of social-cognitive and applied health psychology. Her current research topics include the understanding of drivers of food choice (in particular food avoidance), acceptance of novel technologies in relation to food, and also individual differences with relevance to health attitudes and their impact on (multiple) health behaviours.

Professor Mahinda Abeywardena

Mahinda is a Senior Principal Research Scientist at CSIRO Health and Biosecurity. He has a PhD in pharmacology and over 35 years' experience in nutritional physiology-pharmacology of dietary constituents, including edible oils and fats, long-chain omega-3s and natural bioactives/antioxidants. He has an international reputation in the area of diet, blood vessels and heart health, and was a lead investigator of the team that pioneered the world-first discovery of the preventative properties of fish oil omega-3s in heart health, at a time when fish oil was regarded as a bio-waste. Mahinda has a strong publication record to his credit, serves in the editorial board of several scientific journals and sits on advisory panels on nutrition and in health. He was a co-recipient of the prestigious CSIRO medal for Research Achievement in 2010 for his contributions to produce an alternative plant-based, sustainable source of long-chain omega-3s with enhanced bioavailability.

Introduction

The past decade has seen a sharp increase in scientific research and community interest in the role of the gut in human health. There have been major developments in our understanding of common gut issues such as chronic constipation, bloating and excessive wind, with evidence increasing in the areas of more serious conditions such as irritable bowel syndrome, diverticular disease and colorectal cancer.

Accompanying this growing awareness of how gut health contributes to overall good health, we are starting to unravel more about the gut and its involvement in inflammation, mood and degenerative diseases.

We've long understood the gut's importance as a gateway to our nutrient metabolism, where nutrients and water are extracted from the food we eat to be distributed throughout the body. We also know that fibre slows the absorption of nutrients from our gut, which keeps us feeling fuller for longer and helps regulate our blood sugar. We've also known for a while that the health of the gut is reliant on the health of the huge community of bacteria it sustains.

Newer discoveries are to do with the direct link between the gut and the brain via the nervous system, and that many hormones are released or influenced by the activity of gut bacteria that can affect appetite, sugar metabolism and mood. We also know that gut bacteria play a crucial role in our immune function by keeping our gut wall nourished and strong. Indeed, a condition known as leaky gut is increasingly associated with intestinal diseases, autoimmune disorders and neurological conditions.

Quite simply, our gut health has an enormous impact on our overall health and therefore our quality of life. The explosion of scientific research in this field – with CSIRO at the forefront – has also led to the discovery that feeding our gut bacteria with a particular type of fibre called resistant starch is a major piece in the gut-health puzzle.

Throughout the world, rates of colorectal cancer (commonly known as bowel cancer) and other intestinal conditions such as Crohn's disease, diverticular disease and ulcerative colitis are on the rise. In Australia, bowel cancer is the second most commonly diagnosed cancer (after breast cancer) and the second biggest cancer killer (after lung cancer) with more than 5000 deaths each year. Yet, paradoxically, Australia also has one of the highest intakes of fibre in the Western world which, according to decades of research, should be helping to protect us against bowel cancer. We now know that in Australia at least, this enigma of high-fibre intake and high colon cancer rates can be attributed to our low intake of resistant starch.

This book was written by a team of CSIRO researchers, nutrition and behaviour scientists and dietitians, many of whom are internationally recognised authorities in nutrition and gut health.

Australia is number 8 on the world list for colorectal cancer cases.

Our mission is to encourage all Australians to boost not only their intake of fibre in general (our intake is relatively high, though not high enough) but also their intake of resistant starch. This might sound daunting, but we assure you it's not. In fact, the message is a familiar one: we need to eat a wide variety of whole plant foods (wholegrain cereals, vegetables, fruits, legumes, nuts and seeds).

———————

In Part 1 we explain how the gut functions in concert with our microbiota to promote a healthy metabolism and immune system. We describe the different kinds of fibres (soluble, insoluble and resistant starch) and how they work together to promote a diverse, balanced and resilient microbiota. We also talk about normal digestive function (yes, it's something we all need to be more comfortable discussing) and outline some of the symptoms and treatments for a number of the major gut-related disorders.

———————

In Part 2 we show you exactly what foods you need to eat to amp up your fibre and resistant starch, and include meal plans that can be tailored to your individual needs. There are sample daily plans for people who need to follow a low-FODMAP diet, as well as those diagnosed with wheat or lactose intolerances, to use as a guide in consultation with your healthcare team.

———————

In Part 3 we provide lots of delicious, easy-to-cook recipes that are designed to benefit the gut and overall health. Most contain higher amounts of fibre and resistant starch to feed the gut microbiota. Based on fresh, seasonal wholefoods, the recipes provide a balanced intake of all the important nutrients for good health and are consistent with our core dietary principle of higher proteins and lower carbohydrates.

The CSIRO Healthy Gut Diet is the result of decades of multi-stranded research into the relationship between the gut and other bodily systems, the gut's role in disease and how different foods affect gut health. Yet while the research is complex, the overarching message is beautifully simple. You can dramatically improve your gut health, as well as your overall health and wellbeing, by eating a healthy balanced diet, with plenty of fibre – including resistant starch – and by exercising regularly.

PART ONE

Healthy Gut, Healthy Body

What is *the* gut?

Before we go any further, let's define just what we mean by the word 'gut'. For many people it's a vague term for the mid-section of the body – the stomach and intestines – but in this book we use it to mean the entire gastrointestinal (GI) tract from start to end.

The gut (also called the alimentary canal) can be thought of as one long hollow 'tube' of variable diameter that takes in food at one end and passes waste products out the other. But of course it is much more complex than that. On average the total GI tract (including the oesophagus and stomach) is about 9 metres long, and the intestinal bits are folded repeatedly to fit into our abdominal cavity. The inside of the tube is lined by a continuation of our skin called the epithelium, and the gut cavity, also known as the gut lumen, sits inside this. The epithelium is also highly convoluted, which increases the surface area available for the absorption of nutrients from our food. (In fact, the total surface area is estimated to be somewhere between 30 and 40 square metres – the size of a small room!) The epithelium (the gut mucosa) also secretes a thick mucus that protects the gut from damage, harsh chemicals and pathogenic (disease-causing) bacteria. The lower gut is colonised by a large population of gut microbes (mostly bacteria) known as the gut microbiota.

Anatomically, the gut can be sectioned into five main parts: mouth, oesophagus, stomach, and small and large intestines, as shown in the diagram below. There are also ancillary organs – the liver (and gallbladder) and pancreas which, although technically outside the gut, are directly connected to it by ducts and support its digestive work. The vascular and nervous systems are also integral to gut functions.

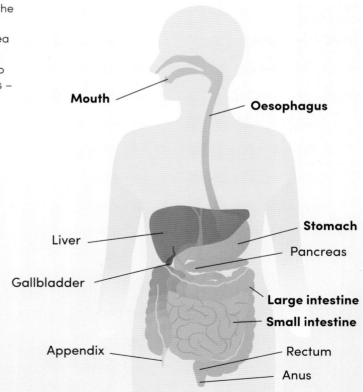

Mouth

Oesophagus

Liver

Stomach

Pancreas

Gallbladder

Large intestine

Small intestine

Appendix

Rectum

Anus

The *mechanics* of digestion

The main job of the gut is to extract essential nutrients from our food and deliver them, and water, to the bloodstream and eventually the tissues of the body. Complex carbohydrates are broken down to glucose; proteins to amino acids; and fats to fatty acids and glycerol. Digestion is a long and intricate process that actually begins when the aroma of food activates our salivary glands, ready for that first mouthful.

The mouth and oesophagus

The first stage of digestion occurs when we chew our food and mix it with saliva. Our saliva contains enzymes called amylases which immediately start to break down the starches in the food.

When we swallow a mouthful of chewed food (called a bolus), it moves into the oesophagus, and a valve called the upper oesophageal sphincter closes behind it. Peristaltic movement – caused by contractions in the muscles of the oesophagus wall in a circular motion – then takes the bolus down to the top of the stomach, where a second valve (the lower oesophageal sphincter) opens to allow the food in, then closes again immediately.

The stomach

The stomach must be sealed off from the rest of the digestive system because its internal environment is extremely acidic. Cells in the stomach epithelium produce hydrochloric acid and other secretions, which are then churned up with the bolus for 90 minutes to 4 hours. The acid starts to break down the proteins in the food, then enzymes called proteases, in particular pepsin, start disassembling them into their component amino acids. Any bacteria that have entered via the mouth can only pass through the stomach alive if they are acid-resistant.

A number of factors influence rates of gastric emptying – that is, how fast or slow your food travels through the stomach. Dietary factors are complex, but broadly speaking some proteins and dietary fats are known to slow the rate of emptying. However, many other variables also have a large impact, including stress, chronic disease, surgical procedures, hormones and even the weather.

When the partially digested food reaches an appropriate consistency, the stomach intermittently releases it into the small intestine via a valve called the pyloric sphincter. Very little food has been absorbed into the bloodstream at this point. The partially digested food is now referred to as chyme.

The small intestine

Also often referred to as the small bowel, the small intestine is very long, highly folded and has an internal surface covered in finger-like projections called villi. It has three main sections, the duodenum, jejunum and ileum.

In the duodenum, the chyme is mixed with bile. (Bile is made in the liver, stored in the gallbladder and enters the intestine via the bile duct.) Bile breaks down fats in our food so that they can be further broken down into their component parts by enzymes called lipases, which are secreted into the duodenum by the pancreas. The juices from the pancreas also contain more amylases to further break down carbohydrates, and more proteases to keep working on the protein in the chyme. Digestive enzymes are also secreted from the epithelium of the intestine.

The chyme then moves into the jejunum, where most nutrient absorption occurs. Nutrients of every kind are transported across the epithelium and into the bloodstream, where they can be transported to cells throughout the body to meet immediate fuel needs, to be used structurally or to be stored for later. In the ileum, what remains of the chyme – which is now largely water and indigestible components – slows down. Here the bacterial population begins to increase. A little more absorption occurs, most notably of vitamin B12 and bile salts, and the chyme then moves into the large intestine.

The large intestine

The large intestine (often referred to as the bowel) consists of the caecum, appendix, colon, rectum and anal canal. The caecum and appendix play relatively minor roles in digestion.

The colon is an important part of the digestion process. It's here that bacteria feed on undigested material through a process called fermentation, producing substances such as short-chain fatty acids that keep epithelial cells lining the bowel healthy. Trace amounts of minerals such as calcium and magnesium are recovered here, and excess water is also absorbed from the colon, which helps to soften stools. Conversely, increased fluid can tend to make stools firm. Although the colon is only 1.6 metres in length, the digestion process in this part of the gut can take up to 30 hours or even longer.

The rectum acts as an assembly point for faeces, which build up until the next bowel movement through the anus. And thus, 24–60 hours after we took our first bite, our food's journey is complete.

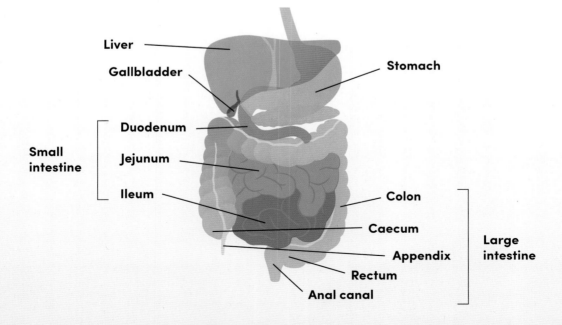

Liver — Stomach

Gallbladder

Duodenum

Small intestine — Jejunum

Ileum — Colon

Caecum

Appendix — Large intestine

Rectum

Anal canal

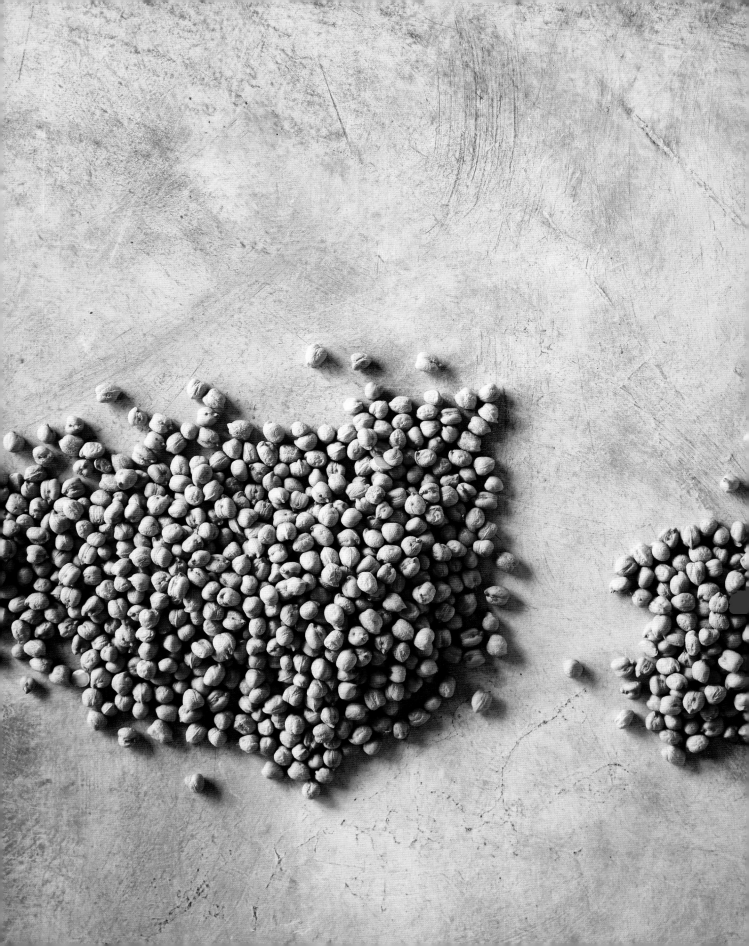

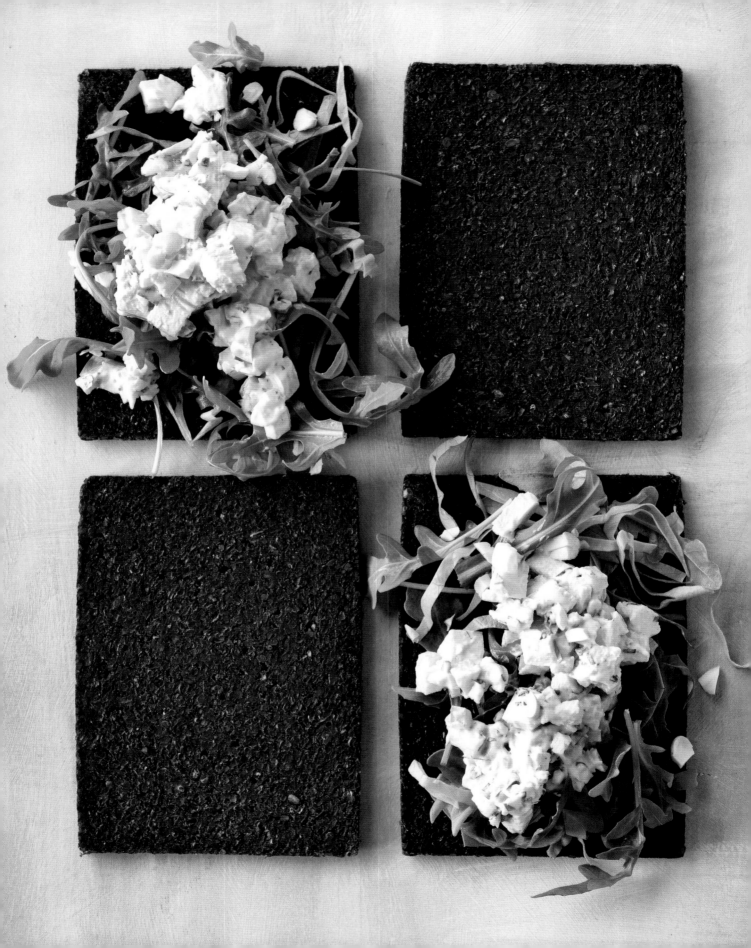

The gut–brain *connection*

The hypothalamus (specifically the arcuate nucleus) is the main part of the brain responsible for energy homeostasis (the regulation of food intake and energy expenditure). Gut hormones are key players in mediating the interaction between the gut and the brain, informing the brain – in particular the hypothalamus and brain stem – about what nutrients are present in the gut (see the box below). These hormonal signals, largely transmitted via the circulation, tell us when our energy stores are running low. They also have a role to play in blood glucose control.

There is also evidence that gut bacteria and their products can affect how our brain functions, and may have a role to play in mood and anxiety. This may be achieved through products reaching circulation, or through effects on the central nervous system (e.g. via the vagus nerve which extends from the brain to the lower GI tract).

Gut hormones are key players in mediating the interaction between the gut and the brain.

UNDERSTANDING GUT HORMONES

Ghrelin is an appetite-stimulating hormone that is mainly produced by the stomach, and is the only gut hormone known to promote food intake. Ghrelin levels naturally increase after fasting or vigorous exercise, telling us to eat so that our body rebuilds its energy levels.

Leptin is a hormone which opposes the actions of ghrelin and helps regulate energy metabolism by inhibiting feelings of hunger. Leptin is mainly produced by cells that store fat and, by signalling the brain to suppress hunger, it helps regulate fat accumulation.

Secretin is released in the small intestine and is important in regulating a number of functions related to digestion. It sends a signal to the brain to regulate water homeostasis in the body, and modulates the pH of the small intestine by inhibiting the release of stomach acids. It also assists in breakdown of fats by stimulating the release of bile.

Cholecystokinin (CCK) is a short-term appetite-suppressing hormone, which is released in the small intestine as we eat both protein and fats, telling the body we have what we need for that meal. It's also involved in the regulation of blood sugar levels, inhibiting glucose production in the liver.

Glucagon-like peptide 1 (GLP1) is a short-term appetite-suppressing hormone produced in the lower part of the small intestine in response to carbohydrates, proteins and fats. It slows the rate of gastric emptying, providing greater glycaemic control.

Peptide YY (PYY) is an appetite-suppressing hormone released in the lowest part of the bowel (ileum, colon and rectum) in direct proportion to the calorie content of a meal. Levels peak after a meal in order to signal fullness to the brain.

Our *gut* microbiota

You'll probably be aware that microscopic organisms (including bacteria, fungi and viruses) are actually found in other areas of the human body as well as the gut: these include the skin, the respiratory tract, urinary tract and vagina.

Our colon supports a large and diverse population of bacteria. These, in turn, provide us with essential micronutrients (e.g. vitamins B and K) and energy-producing metabolites, such as short-chain fatty acids. The bacteria also make use of sloughed intestinal cells and secretions, harvesting the nutrients and energy they contain. Microbial activity also helps in the release and uptake of essential trace elements, such as calcium and magnesium.

Each individual has a unique combination of many hundreds of different types of gut bacteria. While the characteristics of our gut microbial profile are established in the first few years of life and strongly influenced by how we were delivered and whether or not we were breast-fed, the profile does change as we age.

Our microbiota is determined by factors such as diet, the environment, our genes and even our lifestyle. However, sudden adverse shifts in microbial populations (dysbiosis) can occur as a result of disease, infection, antibiotic use or other influences.

Taking antibiotics to treat bacterial infections can upset the microbial balance in our gut and lead to digestive problems. This is why pharmacists may suggest a probiotic (along with a prescribed antibiotic) to help our microbiota re-establish balance.

The impact of long-term dietary patterns on gut microbial profiles is not yet well understood, but we do know that for most people, eating a broad range of whole foods naturally high in fibre is likely to increase the activity and numbers of some of the bacteria that help our gut and our health overall. A study conducted by CSIRO was able to show that most people could boost production of the beneficial microbial product butyric acid in their large bowel by increasing the consumption of resistant starch in their diet.

Probiotics and prebiotics

Popular ways to increase the numbers of beneficial bacteria in the gut is through the consumption of probiotics and prebiotics. **Probiotics** are live bacteria (including many species of *Bifidobacterium* and *Lactobacillus*) that provide a health benefit, and are commonly found in yoghurts and some fermented foods. They can also be consumed in capsule form.

The effectiveness of using probiotics is often debated. Some studies show health benefits while others do not. There are multiple strains of probiotics available and before you select a variety it is recommended that you speak with your health professional. Results may depend on the type of probiotic consumed, the food it may be in, whether there are sufficient numbers of microbes present, and whether it is taken regularly enough. There is now growing recognition that the use of prebiotics may be a better alternative.

Prebiotics are food components that selectively stimulate the growth and activity of certain bacteria, which thereby result in a health benefit. Resistant starch fibre and other dietary fibres such as inulin (present in large amounts in chicory root, and in smaller amounts in garlic, onion, asparagus and bananas) increase numbers of beneficial microbes such as *Bifidobacterium* and are regarded as prebiotics. The advantage of prebiotics is that they stimulate the growth and activity of microbes that would normally already exist within the gut of an individual.

The gut and the *immune system*

Our gut is a frontline of our immune system.

In fact, around 70–80 per cent of the body's immune cells (mucosal-related lymphoid tissue) are found in the gut, which makes sense when you consider that many toxins and pathogenic invaders can enter the body through our digestive system. Our gut then needs to be our first line of defence.

Our immune system also interacts closely with our microbiota, which is important as our bodies need to be able to differentiate between friendly bacteria and any interlopers that can make us sick.

Leaky gut

Although commonly thought to be controversial, research into leaky gut (intestinal permeability) is now becoming more widely accepted and recognised as being important in gut health management. Our immune system has evolved over millennia to prevent pathogenic microorganisms in our gut from entering our body and negatively impacting our health. This protection requires intact tissue along the inner gut wall (the epithelium), and a healthy layer of mucus above it. Although numerous factors contribute to a breakdown in gut-barrier function, our diet plays a significant role.

In a healthy gut, the epithelial cells that line the gut are tightly connected by proteins to form a barrier between the gut and the rest of the body. Any materials that enter the body must pass through the cells themselves via specific channels. We now know, however, that this barrier can be disrupted by a poor diet (one that is low in resistant starch and high in processed foods, salt, sugar and total fats), leading to a condition called increased intestinal permeability, commonly known as leaky gut.

In a leaky gut, the proteins that form the tight connection between the cells become damaged, causing gaps to form between the cells. This means that foreign materials and toxins which normally do not enter the body will 'leak' through the gaps, causing low-level inflammation.

Inflammation occurs when the body attempts to neutralise or eliminate foreign materials. Our tissues release chemical messengers (e.g. inflammatory cytokines) to attract immune cells to eliminate the foreign invaders. Some of the bacteria in the colon produce harmful chemicals known as endotoxins, and if the gut is leaky these can enter the bloodstream, causing inflammation.

Leaky gut has been associated with a wide range of disorders, from intestinal and liver diseases to autoimmune disorders such as type 1 diabetes. Leaky gut is more common among obese people and is believed to contribute to associated conditions such as type 2 diabetes.

There is a new dual sugar intestinal permeability blood test available for the diagnosis of leaky gut. Currently CSIRO researchers are exploring specialised dietary patterns to restore and maintain a healthy gut barrier. A diet high in resistant starch and zinc (see below) will work towards keeping your gut healthy and may prevent or reduce the progression of leaky gut. Speak with your GP or an accredited practising dietitian with experience in managing gut disorders, who can help you repair a leaky gut with a nutrient-dense diet and if needed, weight loss.

Why zinc?

Zinc plays an important role in the growth and development of cells and cell metabolism and as such assists in maintaining and restoring the gastrointestinal mucosal structure. However, since zinc is a mineral and can be toxic in high doses, supplementation needs to be monitored by your dietitian.

Fibre: a *key* to gut health

For many years it was thought that fibre was simply the tough parts of plant foods (roughage) that promoted regularity by bulking up stools. But we now know that many of fibre's health benefits involve our gut microbiota.

Dietary fibre comprises a large, diverse group of mainly indigestible carbohydrates. We get these indigestible compounds largely from plant foods (cereals, vegetables, fruits, legumes, nuts and seeds). 'Indigestible' means that we do not break down these carbohydrates during digestion in the upper gut. As such, fibre gives you much less dietary energy (kilojoules/calories) than digestible carbohydrates.

Most of the microbiota in our gut have enzymes that can break down ('ferment') some of these carbohydrates into short-chain fatty acids. These short-chain fatty acids, in particular butyrate, have several important health benefits.

- They create an environment unfavourable to the growth of pathogens and other potentially harmful microbes.
- They enhance the immune response, reinforcing the gut barrier and the gut mucosa.
- They inhibit inflammation, keeping the bowel cells healthy and helping them recognise and eliminate the DNA mutations that can lead to colorectal cancer (also known as colon cancer or bowel cancer).
- They promote fluid and electrolyte uptake in the large bowel.
- Butyrate is a fuel for the epithelial cells of our large intestine.

Aside from nourishing our microbiome, fibre also has some other important health benefits:

- it enhances the feeling of fullness after a meal and can therefore suppress hunger
- it improves control of blood-sugar levels by stimulating insulin sensitivity.

Types of dietary fibre

Traditionally, fibres have been classified as either insoluble or soluble. Generally, insoluble fibres are represented by 'roughage', which is poorly fermented, whereas soluble fibres are readily utilised by the gut microbiota. But not all fibres fit neatly into this simple classification system. Resistant starch is essentially an insoluble fibre, but behaves more like a soluble fibre – it is readily fermented and a very important food source for gut microbiota (see page 20).

Insoluble fibre

This is the tough stuff – the cell walls, outer skin and structural parts of plants, and accounts for about 70 per cent of most plant food fibre. Insoluble fibre tends to be slowly and incompletely fermented by gut bacteria. The undigested fibre is important because it 'mechanically' stimulates the lining of the gut, helping propel food along the intestinal tract and attracting water to keep stools soft. In this way it helps prevent constipation and other common gut problems.

Insoluble fibres are found in grains, wholegrain cereals, nuts, seeds, fruit and vegetables. Wheat bran is a highly concentrated source of insoluble fibre (only about 30 per cent of wheat bran fibre is fermented completely in the gut), which is why it is often used to treat constipation.

Fibre enhances the feeling of fullness after a meal and can therefore suppress hunger.

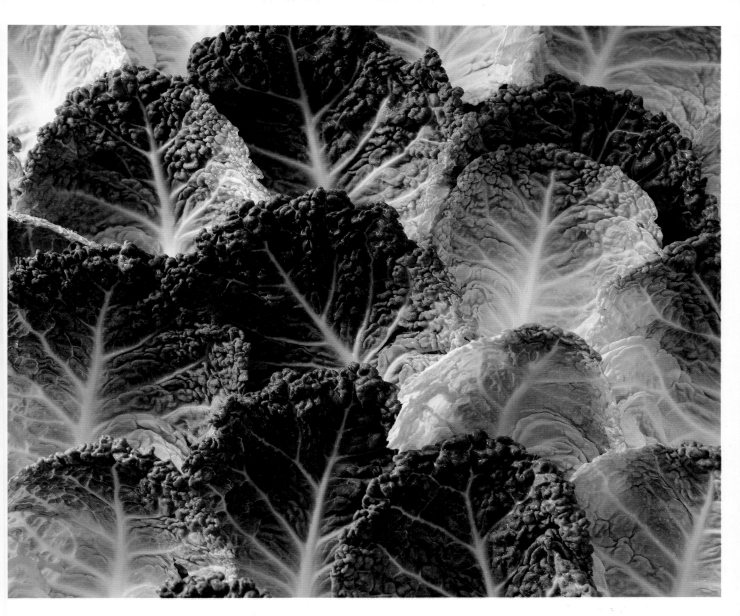

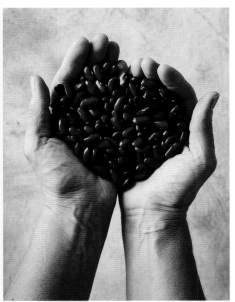

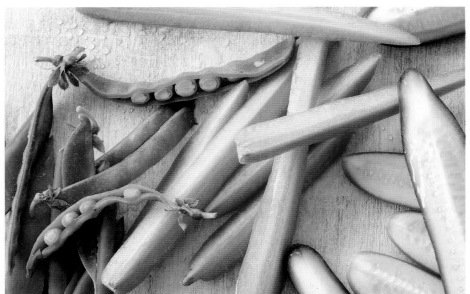

Type of fibre	Key properties	Best food sources
INSOLUBLE	<ul><li>Slowly and only partially fermented</li><li>Retains water</li><li>Increases the volume of food undergoing digestion and faecal bulk</li><li>Improves stool form and aids laxation</li><li>Improves control of blood sugar by stimulating insulin sensitivity</li></ul>	<ul><li>Most **wholegrain foods**, such as wholegrain cereals, bread and pasta</li><li>Fibre-rich cereal, such as **bran**</li><li>**Legumes**, such as beans, chickpeas, lentils, green and yellow split peas</li><li>Most **vegetables**, but especially green peas and beans, spinach, silverbeet (chard), cabbage, broccoli, beetroot, parsnip, carrot and brussels sprouts</li><li>Most **fruit**, but especially unpeeled pears and apples, oranges, passionfruit, figs, strawberries and raspberries</li><li>**Nuts** and **seeds**</li></ul>
SOLUBLE	<ul><li>Highly fermentable</li><li>Supports growth and activity of beneficial bacteria that promote a healthy colonic environment</li><li>Viscous forms are important for heart and metabolic health due to reduced glycaemic response</li></ul>	<ul><li>**Legumes**, **nuts** and **seeds**</li><li>**Psyllium husks**, **oats** and **barley**</li><li>Most **vegetables**, but especially parsnips, okra, brussels sprouts, eggplant, green peas, broad beans, green beans and onions</li><li>**Fruits** such as pears, mango, prunes, apples and oranges</li></ul>
RESISTANT STARCH	<ul><li>Completely fermented</li><li>Encourages growth and activity of bacteria that produce butyrate (a short-chain fatty acid important for the integrity and health of the bowel wall)</li><li>Suppresses populations of potential pathogens</li><li>Important for heart and metabolic health due to reduced glycaemic response</li></ul>	<ul><li>**Wholegrain** bread, millet, puffed flakes, rye and barley</li><li>**Legumes**</li><li>**Cold cooked** starchy foods, such as potatoes, rice, pasta and beans</li><li>**Firm bananas**, green peas and artichokes</li><li>**Novel cereals**, such as BARLEYmax™, high-amylose wheat and high-amylose maize (see page 44)</li></ul>

Soluble fibre

Generally, the more soluble a fibre, the more quickly and more extensively it is fermented by the gut bacteria.

Smaller fibres – such as inulin and other fructans (see FODMAPs on page 34) – are highly soluble and are rapidly fermented to completion (mostly in the first part of the large bowel).

Beta-glucans (found in oats and barley) and pectins (found in legumes, apples and citrus fruits) are of intermediate solubility and are moderately fermentable. They also become viscous (gooey) in solution, which helps slow digestion, and reduce blood glucose and LDL cholesterol levels.

Psyllium is an unusual fibre in that it is soluble but poorly fermented. It has a particularly strong water-holding capacity, which helps with laxation.

Resistant starch

This is the real gold. Unlike other insoluble fibres, resistant starch is preferentially and extensively fermented by our gut bacteria. Most importantly, it is 'butyrogenic' (i.e. its fermentation favours butyrate production), which, as we have seen, has important flow-on effects for gut-wall integrity, healthy digestion and optimal immune function.

While our bodies can easily break down 'ordinary' starch, resistant starch goes through the first part of the digestive system intact. Resistant starch occurs naturally in all starchy foods, but most of the commonly consumed ones, such as potatoes and bakery products, contain minimal amounts. The best sources of resistant starch are legumes and wholegrain cereals.

Resistant starch can also be formed during food production and preparation. If we cook potatoes and allow them to cool before eating them – in a potato salad, say – the structure of the starch changes and there is a *modest* rise in resistant starch content. This process, called retrogradation or staling, used to be common in the days before refrigeration and supermarkets.

How much fibre do we need?

The total daily fibre intake recommended is 25 grams for women and 30 grams for men. These amounts are considered adequate for maintaining gut function and laxation. However, to reduce the risk of chronic diseases, the National Health and Medical Research Council suggests higher daily intakes: 28 grams for women and 38 grams for men.

The importance of fibre diversity

As we have seen, not all fibres are equal. Some are more effective at increasing stool bulk than others, and their susceptibility to fermentation and ability to feed the gut microbiota also differ. Since individual fibres vary greatly in their capacity to promote gut health and function, the best option is to consume a wide variety of whole foods that are as close to their natural state as possible – wholegrain cereals, fruits, vegetables, legumes and a few nuts and seeds. Fibre diversity ensures that fermentation, and the resulting production of short-chain fatty acids (and other protective metabolites) occurs along the entire length of the large bowel and no part misses out.

Resistant starch is the real gold – it promotes gut-wall integrity, healthy digestion and optimal immune function.

Why minimally processed foods are best

Whole plant-based foods (wholegrain cereals, fruits, vegetables, legumes, nuts and seeds) are not only high in fibre, but also bursting with vitamins, minerals and other nutrients. They are also naturally low in salt, sugar and fat.

Whole plant foods retain much of the plant's cell wall structure, which means particles are larger, fermentation is slower and more of the fibre reaches the colon, thus raising resistant starch content.

To help keep the cell wall structure intact:
* avoid pureeing or juicing where possible
* avoid peeling vegetables or fruits where possible
* use coarse bran rather than finely milled bran (if you are needing to use it as a laxative).

Can we have too much fibre?

If you are not used to having much fibre in your diet, a sudden increase may sometimes produce abdominal discomfort and increased flatulence, but these side effects can be minimised by:
* increasing fibre intake gradually, and spreading consumption of high-fibre foods throughout the day (not just at breakfast)
* drinking plenty of water. Fibre needs water as a vehicle to move it along!

Fibre intake is usually self-limiting when wholefoods are consumed, which is why we have not set an upper intake level for vegetables (see page 50).

Will I put on weight?

Fibre has half the kilojoules of digestible carbohydrates and incompletely fermented fibres have even less, so fibre is not associated with weight gain. In fact, it is associated with a sense of fullness and therefore can reduce the risk of overeating.

Whole plant foods retain much of the plant's cell wall structure, which means fermentation is slower, thus raising resistant starch content.

Is my gut *healthy?*

A healthy gut digests and absorbs food efficiently and effectively, removes water from waste for use by the body, and eliminates waste products appropriately.

Basically, it does its job 24/7 without us noticing, except for a rumbling belly, gas and the occasional bout of extra-firm or runny stools. What's abnormal is to have consistent pain, recurrent constipation or diarrhoea, troublesome and/or painful gas, or blood in the stool. Most gut problems are benign and involve the large intestine, but the early symptoms of serious, life-threatening problems are often difficult to distinguish from harmless disorders, so any persistent gut ailments should be discussed with your doctor.

So what are the markers of healthy gut function?

Gas

Regularly passing gas (out of either end) is a sign that your gut is functioning normally. Remember that your gut microbes are fermenting, which by definition involves the production of gas – which has to escape somehow. If circumstances don't permit the free escape of gas, it may lead to subsequent bloating and cramping. Some people may be more sensitive to bowel wall distension than others. A healthy adult passes about 0.5 to 1.5 litres of flatus daily. The total volume is about the same regardless of gender, but the number of events is greater for men than women, about 12 and 8, respectively.

Bowel habits

Bowel habit is another good marker of how well your gut is generally functioning. How often you pass a bowel movement, and what is passed into the bowl, offers an insight into your gut's state of health.

Frequency and transit time

Bowel habits vary greatly among adults, with 'normal' frequency ranging anywhere from three times a day to three times a week. (As a side note, the frequency tends to be greater in babies, especially those that are breast-fed, and less in the elderly.)

The rate at which food moves though the gut is known as transit time. Transit time is a determinant of faecal weight, and very slow transit times are associated with low faecal weights. Epidemiological studies have shown that slower transit times, and lower faecal weights, are associated with greater risk of developing gut diseases and disorders.

Transit time, although determined largely by our genetics, is strongly influenced by our intake of dietary fibre. Other factors include exercise, fluid intake, mood, hormones, medications and changes in daily routine.

It's also important to 'go when you need to go'. If you feel the urge, but resist (for whatever reason), this may cause you to become constipated.

Stool consistency

Regularly passing a soft, formed stool at a suitable frequency that does not involve urgency, straining or lasting discomfort would seem ideal for most people. Stools should be light to deep brown, smooth and cylindrical, and not hard, lumpy or flattened (see Appendix page 216).

When to see a doctor

A sustained change in bowel habit involving pain or discomfort should not be ignored. Take note of your symptoms and see your doctor. It is important that you do not self-treat as this may make things worse.

Severe, prolonged or recurring pain requires medical evaluation. Stools that are black or light coloured (greyish), or show signs of blood or mucus, necessitate investigation by your doctor.

Consult your doctor immediately if you notice blood in faeces or vomit, if there is unintended or unexplained weight loss, or you have difficulty swallowing. For malignant and other serious bowel diseases, there may be no early symptoms and if there are, they are often difficult to distinguish from non-life-threatening disorders.

About 50 per cent of
Australians report having
experienced problems with
their gut in the past year.

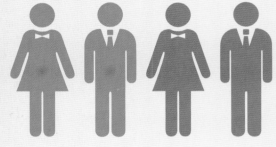

Gut *problems*

Our rates of various conditions associated with the gut – such as colorectal cancer, inflammatory bowel disease and irritable bowel syndrome – are rising, which as we have seen may be associated with gut microbial dysbiosis and leaky gut.

About 50 per cent of Australians report having experienced problems with their gut in the past year. While many factors may be responsible, a diet high in processed foods and low in dietary fibre is often a key contributor. Lack of exercise, obesity, stress, smoking and excessive alcohol consumption are also factors that can negatively impact gut health.

Obesity

Obesity may contribute to gut problems such as leaky gut and inflammation. Obesity arises from a long-term positive energy balance. This means that on average those who are carrying more weight are eating more than their body requires. Other factors, including genetics and environment, do have an impact on weight, though to a lesser extent.

Sweetened beverages, fried foods, cakes and pastries are high in added sugar, saturated fats and low in fibre. These foods are not only commonly associated with obesity, but are also dramatically linked with other conditions including type 2 diabetes and heart disease, which in turn are characterised by long-term, low-grade inflammation (a key characteristic of the overweight and obese).

Dietary macronutrients, apart from differing in their energy densities and glycaemic index profiles – generally fat provides double the energy of protein and carbohydrates – also have different effects on satiety (whether or not we feel full after a meal). Protein is the most satiating macronutrient, therefore diets with a higher protein content compared to diets higher in fat and refined carbohydrates can help to control the overconsumption of total dietary energy, thereby protecting against weight gain. Carbohydrates are next in the hierarchy of satiating macronutrients, while fats have been reported as the least satiating. In support of this, studies show that obese individuals over-consume energy when exposed to a high-fat meal compared to a meal high in carbohydrates.

Importantly, dietary fibre may influence appetite, energy intake and body weight. Foods high in fibre often require more chewing, thus allowing more time for the release of satiety signals. Furthermore, some dietary fibre such as soluble fibres (e.g. beta-glucan) can increase nutrient retention time in the stomach and intestines, thereby reducing the amount of food consumed at subsequent meals and throughout the day. Finally, once fermentable fibres reach the large intestine they are fermented by gut bacteria, generating short-chain fatty acids which can influence satiety by promoting the release of gut hormones, that directly signal to regions of the brain involved with satiety (e.g. the hypothalamus).

Coeliac disease

Coeliac disease is a food hypersensitivity caused by an immune response to gluten. The body attacks the intestines themselves, causing serious damage to the gut. This makes coeliac disease an autoimmune condition. It cannot be cured, and the only treatment is a completely gluten-free diet for life.

Many people now favour a gluten-free diet, but only those with coeliac disease need to adopt this diet. People who have a sensitivity to gluten can actually eat small amounts without suffering symptoms. In some cases, their sensitivity may not actually be to the gluten in wheat, but to other substances wheat contains, called fructans (or fructo-oligosaccharides). For these people, a low-FODMAP approach can be the best solution – the 'O' in FODMAP stands for oligosaccharides (see page 34). As with all intestinal conditions, it is important to consult your doctor.

Food allergies and intolerances

There has been a growing public interest in food allergies and intolerances in more recent years – and having access to a wide range of less-than-robust 'scientific' information has caused a lot of confusion.

Many people with gut symptoms, such as bloating or general discomfort and gas, have a tendency to diagnose themselves with having one or another food intolerance and will start to avoid particular types of food, such as wheat or dairy – but the culprit for their symptoms may not always be the one they thought.

There is a vast range of possible negative responses to food, from abdominal discomfort to life-threatening anaphylaxis.

Food allergies occur when a particular substance in a food triggers an immune response that causes the body to produce antibodies. Chemicals released as part of this immune response can cause various symptoms throughout the body, in severe cases leading to anaphylactic shock and, if not appropriately managed, death. The best known of these is peanut allergy. **Coeliac disease** is also an immune response to a substance in food (the gluten in wheat), but the symptoms occur mainly in the gut and are slower-acting.

Food intolerances are responses to a food that don't involve the immune system. They do cause abdominal symptoms, headache and fatigue, but do no physical damage, although they can affect a person's quality of life. Food intolerances are commonly dose-dependent, which means that small amounts of the food can be eaten without causing symptoms. However, larger proportions or a frequent intake of the trigger food can mean the person's symptoms can worsen even with small amounts (i.e. reaching their tolerance threshold). The best known of these is **irritable bowel syndrome** (see pages 32–33) triggered by FODMAP foods (see page 35). It is important to note, however, that not all IBS symptoms are improved by a low-FODMAP diet.

Non-coeliac gluten sensitivity

Currently 1% of the population are diagnosed with coeliac disease (and many go undiagnosed). However, a related condition known as non-coeliac gluten sensitivity has been suggested to affect as much as 10% of the population. These people exhibit symptoms such as gut or skin issues said to be immune responses activated by gluten and other wheat proteins. Currently there are no clinically reliable tests for diagnosing individuals affected by this sensitivity. Reliance on a broad range of symptoms possibly provoked by gluten- and wheat-containing foods remains the current process of identification for our healthcare professionals.

Inflammatory bowel disease

Inflammatory bowel disease (IBD) is caused by chronic (long-term) inflammation of the gut. There are two main types:

1 ulcerative colitis, which is more common and affects only the large intestine
2 Crohn's disease, which is rarer and can affect any part of the gut.

People can have a genetic predisposition to these diseases, but diet and lifestyle are also involved. Both are uncommon in countries where processed foods aren't eaten. We know that gut bacteria, possibly through dysbiosis, are involved in both forms.

It's possible that the ulceration of the lower gut seen in ulcerative colitis is due to an insufficient supply of short-chain fatty acids from resistant starch. It can occur after taking antibiotics, which can kill the gut bacteria, including those that make short-chain fatty acids. Although a high-fibre diet is known to lower the risk of developing ulcerative colitis, treating it by increasing fibre intake in general has yielded little or no improvement.

So far no benefit has been found by increasing fibre after Crohn's disease has developed. Treatment can involve anti-inflammatory drugs, and even surgery to remove severely affected regions of the gut.

Colorectal cancer

Globally, bowel cancer kills more than 600,000 people every year, 5000 of them Australian. In fact, Australia and New Zealand have the highest rates of colorectal cancer in the world. Around 25–30 per cent of colon cancers can be attributed to genetic factors; the remainder are the result of diet and lifestyle factors. It's more common in developed countries where people follow a Western-style diet. The risk factors for colorectal cancer include:

* a family history of the disease
* age – this is the highest risk factor; the incidence of colon cancer increases rapidly over the age of 50
* insufficient fibre – about 18 per cent of these cancers in Australia are due to insufficient fibre intake
* being overweight or obese – this accounts for 9 per cent of colorectal cancers in Australia
* eating an unbalanced diet, particularly one that is low in fibre and high in red and processed meats, with excess alcohol
* smoking – which may interact with alcohol consumption to increase risk further
* insufficient exercise.

Bowel cancer occurs in the lining of the large intestine and is found mainly at the lower end, in the descending colon and rectum. The development from initial small growths called polyps to cancer is slow and takes 10–15 years. Early detection and removal of polyps will prevent them developing into cancer which, if untreated, will spread to other parts of the body. The earlier polyps or cancer are detected, the better the chance of a cure. The disease may be symptom-free for many years but traces of blood may still be detected in the stool (see screening page 32). Or there may be obvious symptoms including visible blood in the stool, gastrointestinal pain and altered bowel habit.

Reducing the risk of colorectal cancer

A 2018 report by the World Cancer Research Foundation identifies that to reduce the risk of colorectal cancer, you should:

* undertake regular physical activity – at least 200 minutes a week of brisk walking or its equivalent, and also stand up regularly if you sit for hours at a time

- maintain a healthy weight
- limit your alcohol consumption
- limit fast foods
- limit sugar-sweetened beverages
- eat cooked wholegrains, fruit, vegetables, legumes and resistant-starch foods.

It has recently been found that in addition to consuming foods high in dietary fibre as listed above, the consumption of dairy products may also lead to a reduction in risk of colorectal cancer. Although no absolute amount has been confirmed, having your three serves of dairy each day will be a good start to balancing your dietary intake in a positive way.

Bowel cancer screening

Because bowel cancer rates are so high in Australia, the government has established the National Bowel Cancer Screening Program to help people detect bowel cancer early. The program uses the faecal occult blood test, which detects blood in stools. Testing kits are sent at regular intervals to all Australians between the ages of 50 and 74. Those whose test is positive are encouraged to arrange a colonoscopy to search for polyps. In this procedure, a doctor inserts a flexible telescope, called an endoscope, into the large intestine and carefully examines the inner surface. The endoscope also houses surgical instruments the doctor can use to operate during the procedure, to remove polyps, cauterise bleeding, collect biopsy samples and so on. Capturing the disease early is critical and results in better outcomes.

Diverticular disease

Diverticular disease is a condition that affects the lining of the large intestine (large bowel), and its incidence increases with age. Only a quarter of those with diverticular disease develop symptoms.

The common cause of diverticular disease is a low fibre intake. A diet low in fibre increases your constipation risk, and with constipation stools are firmer and harder, requiring more pressure to push them along the descending colon. Over time, this increased pressure in the bowel can lead to the development of small pockets in the colon that distend under the pressure (diverticula). When the diverticula become inflamed or infected, this is known as diverticulitis.

Common symptoms include lower abdominal cramps (on the left side of the abdomen), loose bowels or constipation. These symptoms can range in severity from mild to severe, and an assessment by your GP is recommended.

When a person has diverticulitis (inflamed diverticular disease), treatment to clear the infection and inflammation is required to relieve the symptoms. Often treatment will require a low-fibre diet and/or antibiotics under the guidance of your GP and dietitian. As the symptoms and inflammation begin to settle, it is advised that fibre is re-introduced into the diet slowly and symptoms are monitored. To help prevent development of the disease, or future bouts of diverticulitis, it is recommended that a diet high in fibre (with plenty of water) and regular exercise are maintained for good bowel health.

Irritable bowel syndrome

Irritable bowel syndrome (IBS) is a functional gastrointestinal disorder, which means that it causes a variety of abdominal symptoms, but produces no detectable physical changes in the gut itself. Symptoms include abdominal pain and discomfort, constipation and/or diarrhoea, bloating and gas, heartburn, nausea and tiredness. To be diagnosed with IBS your symptoms must have occurred at least once a week in the previous three months, lasted for at least six months, and involve diarrhoea or constipation or a mixture of both. IBS affects about 20 per cent of Australians, and more women than men.

What causes IBS?

Functional gastrointestinal disorders have been associated with problems with abnormal muscle contractions in the gut, hypersensitivity to gut pain, and disrupted communication between the brain and the gut. The gut microbiota of some people with IBS has higher numbers of bacteria that produce different gases or a greater volume of gas. The altered microbiota may also disrupt the immune system in the lining of the gut, causing inflammation and changes in the way the nerves and muscles of the gut function. Up to half of people with IBS first develop their symptoms after an infection (such as gastroenteritis), a round of medication (particularly antibiotics), certain foods (an undiagnosed food intolerance) and/or inflammation, each of which can disrupt the microbial balance.

Treatment for IBS

The treatment of functional gastrointestinal disorders depends on the symptoms. Medications are used to treat abdominal pain and bloating, abnormal movement through the gut and hypersensitivity. Antidepressants are also often prescribed for their beneficial effects, reducing the intensity of chronic gastrointestinal pain and normalising movement through the gut. Probiotics can sometimes be used to treat abdominal pain, but there's limited evidence that they work, and it's unclear which bacterial strains help.

Increased fibre intake has been recommended as a treatment for IBS for many years, but insoluble fibre (such as bran) can actually make pain and bloating worse. Some studies have shown that the fibre intake of people with IBS is the same or higher than the fibre intake of those without it. A 2017 review published in the New England Journal of Medicine did find, however, that psyllium husk was beneficial.

The low-FODMAP diet (pages 34–35), which determines and removes fibre components that cause abdominal symptoms, is helpful for as many as 50–82 per cent of IBS sufferers. Although a popular diet for IBS management, a low-FODMAP diet is not recommended for asymptomatic people. This is because removing FODMAPs from your diet may have negative consequences for bowel health in the long term.

A low-FODMAP diet must be carefully managed – it should not be followed without consulting with your healthcare team.

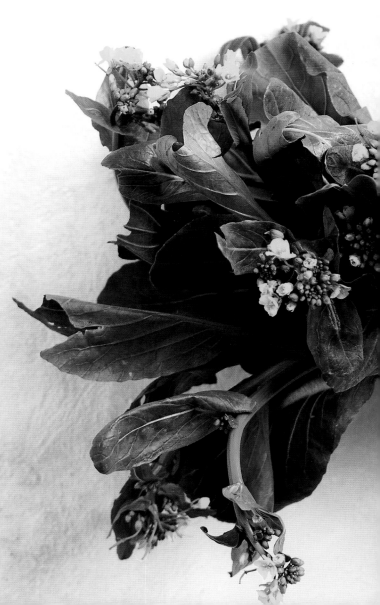

The low-FODMAP diet

FODMAP is an acronym for a group of poorly absorbed carbohydrates (sugars) in food. The low-FODMAP diet is used in clinical practice under the guidance and instruction of trained health professionals and may assist in alleviating gut symptoms. To provide you with some background on the complexities of the diet, we have included a basic overview, including a list of foods that are considered high-FODMAP. For more information on FODMAPs, speak to your GP or a dietitian.

Fermentable – broken down by the gut microbiota
Oligosaccharides – fructans and galacto-oligosaccharides (GOS)
Disaccharides – lactose
Monosaccharides – fructose (in excess of glucose)
And
Polyols – sorbitol, mannitol, xylitol and maltitol

For some individuals, FODMAPs are poorly absorbed in the small intestine, and when they enter the colon are rapidly fermented by bacteria, producing gas. In some people this creates unpleasant symptoms characteristic of irritable bowel syndrome (IBS), including bloating, pain, flatulence, constipation and/or diarrhoea.

We understand that some of our readers may already be progressing on a low-FODMAP diet (under the supervision of their healthcare team) for the management of their professionally diagnosed IBS symptoms. For this reason, we have taken the care to incorporate a low-FODMAP flag in our recipes to guide your choices. As each individual digests FODMAPs differently, we encourage you to discuss the use of these recipes with your healthcare team so that you are getting the most from your diet.

HIGH-FODMAP FOODS

Excess fructose	Fructans	Lactose	GOS	Polyols
Apples	Custard apples	Custard	Chickpeas	Apples
Boysenberries	Nectarines	Condensed milk	Legume beans	Apricots
Figs	White peaches	Dairy desserts	(e.g. baked	Blackberries
Mangoes	Persimmons	Evaporated milk	beans, kidney	Longon
Pears	Tamarillos	Ice cream	beans, borlotti	Lychee
Tamarillos	Watermelon	Milk	beans)	Nashi pears
Watermelon	Artichokes	Milk powder	Lentils	Nectarines
Asparagus	Chicory	Unripened	Cashews	Peaches
Artichokes	Garlic (and	cheese	Pistachio nuts	Pears
Sugar snap peas	powder)	(e.g. ricotta,		Plums
Fruit juices	Leek	cottage cheese,		Cauliflower
Dried fruit	Onion (and	cream cheese,		Mushrooms
High-fructose	powder)	mascarpone)		Snow peas
corn syrup	Spring onions	Yoghurt		Isomalt (953)
Honey	(white part)			Maltitol (965)
	Barley			Mannitol (421)
	Rye			Sorbitol (420)
	Wheat			Xylitol (967)

The CSIRO Healthy Gut Diet includes high fibre, low-FODMAP recipes and a daily sample menu featuring low-FODMAP foods. Please discuss longer-term management of a low-FODMAP diet with your healthcare team, as some of these foods may be re-introduced safely back into your diet under supervision.

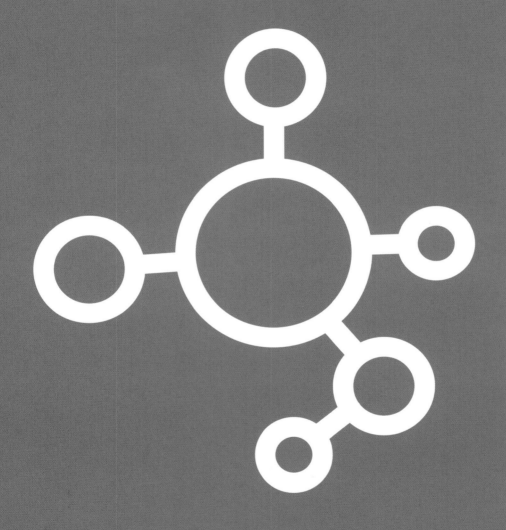

PART TWO

The CSIRO Healthy Gut Eating Plan

Increasing your *fibre* intake

As we saw in Part 1, dietary fibre (and resistant starch in particular) plays a crucial role in supporting, restoring and building a healthy gut microbiota, which in turn furnishes us with nutrients that keep our gut wall healthy and helps reduce the risk of bowel-related disease. **The recommended daily fibre intake for adults is 25 g for women and 30 g for men.**

We also learned that not all fibres are created equal and the best way to ensure we have the right mix of soluble/insoluble fibre and resistant starch is to eat a wide variety of vegetables, legumes and fruit, and to stick to minimally processed wholegrain foods. This table shows you how much fibre is contained in common foods, to help give you a feel for the fibre content of different ingredients.

THE FIBRE CONTENT OF COMMON FOODS

Food	Serving size	Fibre (grams)	CSIRO units
Lean meat, fish, poultry, eggs, tofu			
Beef fillet	100 g (raw)	0	1 unit protein
Chicken breast	100 g (raw)	0	
Fish	100 g (raw)	0	
Eggs	2	0	
Legumes (cooked)	150 g	11 g	
Tofu	170 g	6 g	
Wholegrain breads and cereals			
Sourdough bread	1 slice	2.5 g	1 unit wholegrain breads and cereals (aim for 3 units a day)
Rye bread	1 slice	2.8 g	
Wholemeal bread	1 slice	2.4 g	
Wholegrain crisp bread, e.g. Ryvita	2	2.9 g	
Potato (Carisma)	1 medium	1.7 g	
Legumes	100 g	6 g	
2 Weet-Bix, multigrain	30 g	3.5 g	
BARLEYmax™ (see page 44)	30 g	6 g	
Quinoa (cooked)	½ cup	1.9 g	
Wholemeal pasta (cooked)	½ cup	4.4 g	
Rolled oats	30 g	3.5 g	
Green banana flour	20 g	2.4 g	
Chickpea flour	20 g	2.1 g	
Freekeh, dried	20 g	3.3 g	

THE FIBRE CONTENT OF COMMON FOODS

Food	Serving size	Fibre (grams)	CSIRO units
Dairy			
Milk (1% fat)	250 ml	0	1 unit dairy
Yoghurt	200 g	0.5 g	(aim for 3 units a day)
Cheddar cheese	25 g	0	
Fruit			
Banana	1 large, 150 g	2.7 g	1 unit fruit
Pink Lady apple	1 medium	3.9 g	(aim for 2 units a day)
Blackberries	30 (150 g)	9.2 g	
Nectarine	1 medium	3 g	
Strawberries	12 medium	3.6 g	
Vegetables			
Asparagus	1 cup	3.1 g	1 unit vegetables
Bok choy	1 cup	2 g	(aim for 5 units a day)
Broccoli	1 cup	3.4 g	
Brussels sprouts	1 cup	4.2 g	
Carrot	1 cup	4.6 g	
Cauliflower	1 cup	3.2 g	
Corn	1 cup	9.8 g	
Eggplant	1 cup	2.1 g	
Mushroom	1 cup	1.2 g	
Green peas (cooked)	½ cup	5 g	
Rocket	1 cup	1.3 g	
Spinach	1 cup	1.8 g	
Tomato	1 medium	1.8 g	
Healthy fats and oils			
Extra virgin olive oil	1 teaspoon	0	1 unit healthy
Avocado	20 g	0.6 g	fats and oils
Cashews, almonds and pistachios	7 g	1 g	(aim for 4 units a day)
Indulgences			
Dark chocolate	20 g	0.2 g	1 unit
Red wine	150 ml	0	(limit to 9 units a week)

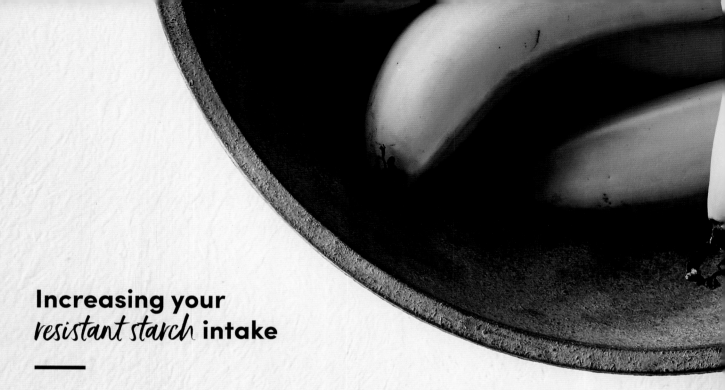

Increasing your *resistant starch* intake

You'll notice in the table on pages 38–39 that we don't list the proportion of resistant starch found in various foods. This is because the exact amount can vary with processing methods, cooking time and temperature, storage and reheating.

Fortunately, we do know which foods contain the highest levels of resistant starch: firm, green (slightly unripe) bananas, beans such as red kidney, lima, adzuki and black-eyed, chickpeas, lentils, green peas, rolled oats (uncooked), white and brown rice and wholemeal pasta (cooked and cooled). We also know that the greater the variety of plant foods we eat, the more resistant starch we will be consuming.

By following the recipes and eating plan in this book you will ensure your diet contains optimum levels of fibre and resistant starch. Here are some additional tips.

- If you are time-poor, use low-salt canned chickpeas, lentils and kidney beans rather than dried. The resistant starch levels are similar in both, but it can take literally hours to prepare the dried versions, whereas canned ones are obviously ready to use straight away.
- When you buy bananas, select slightly under-ripe bananas and eat them within a couple of days. As bananas ripen and turn yellow, the resistant starch content decreases.
- Keep frozen green peas in your freezer, ready to add to curries, stews, soups and stir-fries.
- Experiment with newer high-resistant starch foods on the market such as freekeh, which is made from young durum wheat that has been roasted and rubbed to remove the husk, then cracked (like bulgur). Use it as you would 1 unit of rice.
- Or try thickening a curry, soup or sauce with a flour high in resistant starch, such as chickpea flour or potato starch (not to be confused with potato flour).
- Keep it simple: avoid over-processing your foods to keep the fibre intact.

Shopping tips

Most resistant starch foods can be purchased at supermarkets, your local markets or greengrocer.

- Start in the fresh produce section for green bananas, fruit, vegetables and cashews.
- You can buy dried legumes in bulk from wholesalers, co-ops and whole-food stores, which can work out even cheaper.
- Some products might be harder to find – potato starch and chickpea flour are available in bigger supermarkets, whole-food stores and online. Green banana flour and freekeh are available online, and from some whole-food stores.

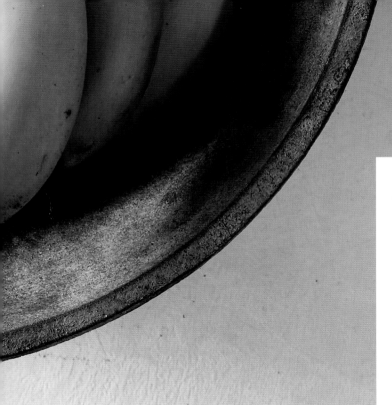

How to prep foods to maximise the amount of resistant starch

Cooking starchy foods like potatoes and rice, then letting them cool overnight and consuming them the next day marginally increases the amount of resistant starch they contain (see page 25). Here are general prep instructions for the most commonly used ingredients in this book:

- ❋ **Potatoes** Steam the diced/chopped potato (or whole potatoes if small) in a steamer basket over a saucepan of simmering water until tender when pierced with a skewer. Cool slightly, then immediately transfer to an airtight container and refrigerate overnight.
- ❋ **Sweet potatoes** Steam the diced/chopped potato in a steamer basket over a saucepan of simmering water until tender. Cool slightly, then immediately transfer to an airtight container and refrigerate overnight.
- ❋ **Rice (for dinnertime quantities of 1 cup/ 185 g cooked rice)** Place ½ cup (100 g) uncooked basmati rice and ¾ cup (180 ml) water in a heavy-based saucepan and bring to the boil over high heat. Cover and reduce the heat to low, then cook for 12 minutes or until all the water has been absorbed and the rice is tender. If you are using brown rice, increase the cooking time to 25–30 minutes. Cool slightly, then immediately transfer to an airtight container and refrigerate overnight.
- ❋ **Rice (for lunchtime quantities of 2 cups /370 g cooked rice)** Place 1 cup (200 g) uncooked basmati rice and 2 cups (500 ml) water in a heavy-based saucepan and bring to the boil over high heat. Cover and reduce the heat to low, then cook for 12 minutes or until all the water has been absorbed and the rice is tender. If you are using brown rice, increase the cooking time to 25–30 minutes. Cool slightly, then immediately transfer to an airtight container and refrigerate overnight.

Food Safety

To decrease the risk of contamination and food poisoning, care needs to be taken with leftover ingredients. Ensure you cool cooked foods quickly; foods left at room temperature for long periods of time may become contaminated. Leftovers need to be stored at 5° or cooler, i.e. in your fridge or freezer, and reheated thoroughly before consumption. Store leftovers in single portions for more efficient cooling and reheating. See foodstandards.gov.au for information on how long specific foods keep for in the fridge or freezer.

Foods containing *resistant starch*
—

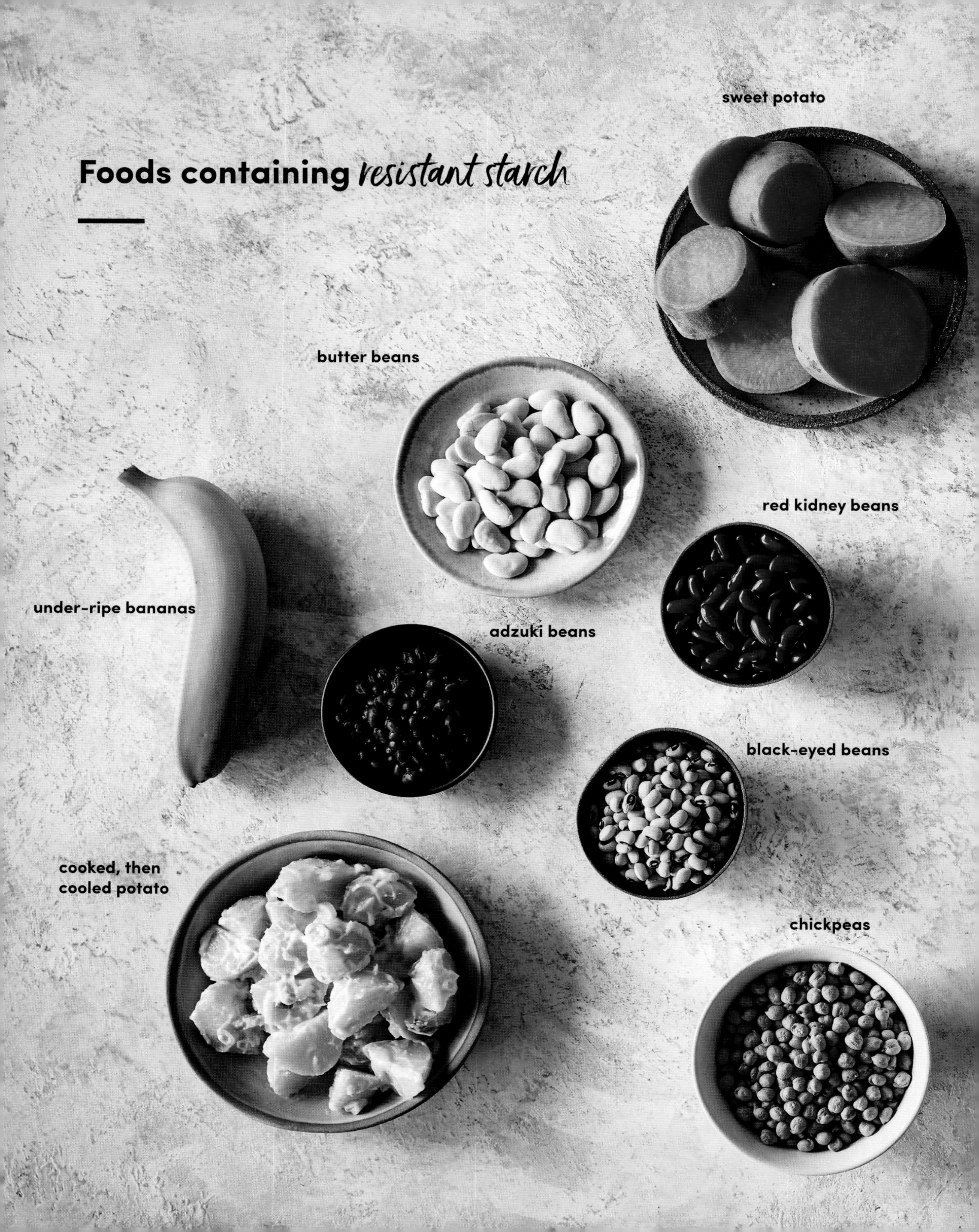

sweet potato

butter beans

red kidney beans

under-ripe bananas

adzuki beans

black-eyed beans

cooked, then
cooled potato

chickpeas

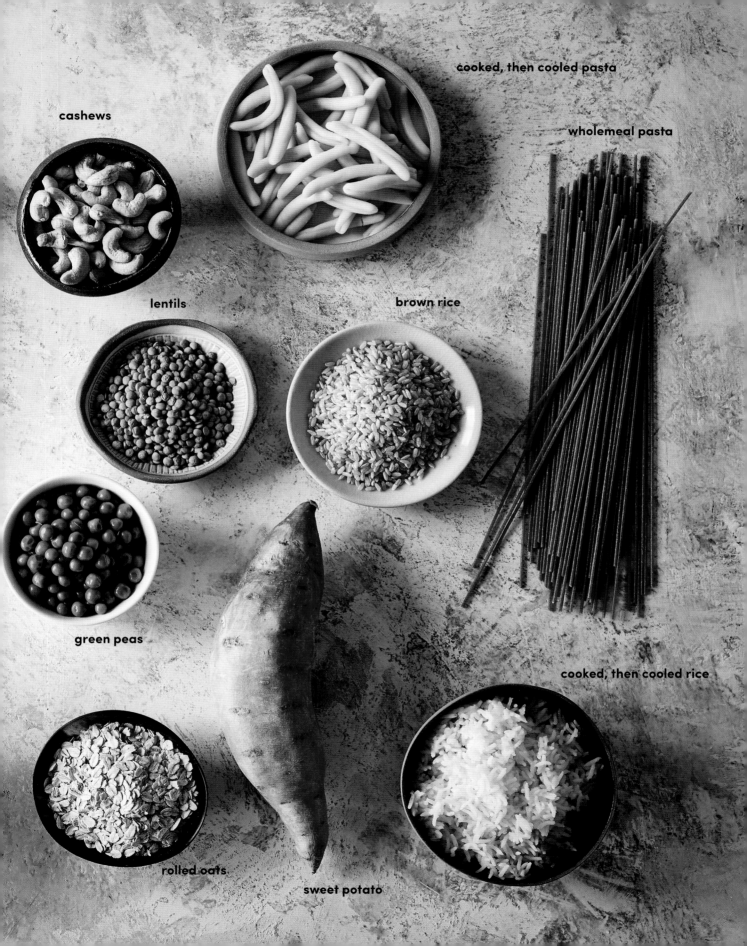

cashews

cooked, then cooled pasta

wholemeal pasta

lentils

brown rice

green peas

cooked, then cooled rice

rolled oats

sweet potato

Increasing your fibre intake with novel grains

CSIRO researchers have found that Australians are just not reaching the daily fibre target of 25–30 grams per day. This is partly due to our preference for refined cereals and our relatively low intake of vegetables and fruits.

To better meet the fibre and health needs of contemporary Australians, CSIRO has been researching ways to increase the resistant starch levels in wheat, barley, rice and other important cereals.

Some of the resulting cereals contain more than twice the total fibre content, and almost ten times the amount of resistant starch. BARLEYmax™ is the first of the new fibre-enriched 'novel' grains developed by CSIRO, and has been formulated into a wide range of healthier foods that are already available in some Australia supermarkets, as well as overseas. Other grains designed by CSIRO to help consumers fill the fibre quantity and quality gap are listed in the table below.

FIBRE-ENRICHED CEREALS DEVELOPED BY CSIRO

Cereal	Nutritional advantage
BARLEYmax™	Very high in several types of fibre
High-amylose wheat	High in resistant starch
Kebari barley	Ultra-low gluten (<5 ppm), high in fibre
High-beta-glucan wheat	High in soluble fibre
High-fructan barley	High in fructans, which are readily fermentable soluble fibres
High-amylose rice	High in resistant starch

High-fibre fruit
___

apples

bananas

We need to reach
a daily fibre target of
25–30 grams per day.

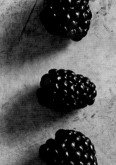

blackberries

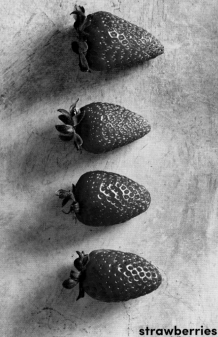

strawberries

peaches

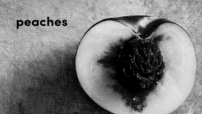

The *Healthy Gut* Eating Plan

Although we are focusing on dietary fibre, which predominantly comes from wholegrains and other plant-based foods, we have taken great care to formulate an eating plan that provides a balanced intake of all the important nutrients for good health and is consistent with our core dietary principle of higher proteins and lower carbohydrates.

The table opposite shows the range of units you will need to consume for each food group in order to obtain the right amount of fibre, essential nutrients and energy **for a 6500 kJ intake**, and is suitable for you if you have a sedentary or inactive lifestyle (i.e. you have a desk job or are driving or sitting and reading most of the day) with very low physical activity levels (mostly walking).

If you are more active, or are not wanting to lose weight, add **1 unit Lean meat, fish, poultry, legumes, eggs and tofu** and **1 unit Wholegrain high-fibre breads and cereals** to each day, keeping in mind you can also have more vegetables across the day.

Improving your gut health is also about maintaining adequate hydration. By increasing your vegetable intake and meeting the unit requirements for each day, you will already be adding more water from foods. However, it is still important to drink at least 3–4 glasses of water or low-calorie fluids every day!

Managing hunger

If you are changing your diet quite considerably, you may feel the urge to eat more. If this is the case, add extra vegetables to your soups, casseroles, salads and snacks (see the 'eat freely' foods list on page 50) to boost the fibre and volume of your meals.

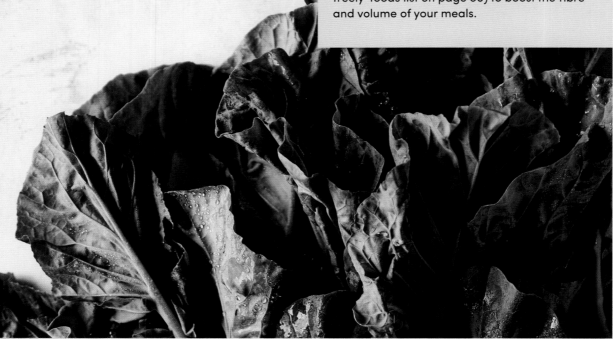

RECOMMENDED DAILY UNITS FOR EACH FOOD GROUP AND AVERAGE NUTRIENT CONTENT PER UNIT

Food group	No. of daily units	Average macronutrient content per unit					
	Based on a 6500 kJ plan	Fibre	Energy	Protein	Carbs	Fat	Comments
Wholegrain high-fibre breads and cereals	3	5 g	400–500 kJ	3 g	15 g	<1 g	Avoid those high in sugar
Lean meat, fish, poultry, eggs, tofu	3	<1 g	500–600 kJ	20 g	0 g	5 g	
Fruit	2	3 g	250–350 kJ	2 g	15 g	0 g	
Vegetables	5	3 g	200–300 kJ	3.5 g	4.5 g	1 g	
Dairy	3	<1 g	500–600 kJ	9 g	9 g	4.5 g	Look for those with no added sugar
Healthy fats and oils	4	0 g	125–200 kJ	0 g	0 g	5 g	
Indulgence foods	Limit to 9 units across the week (less if weight loss is desired)	Limited	450 kJ	Variable	Variable (usually high in added sugar)	Variable (usually high in added fat)	

PORTIONS/QUANTITIES PER UNIT

Food group	1 unit
Wholegrain high-fibre breads and cereals (3 units a day)	❋ 1 slice (40 g) wholegrain bread (e.g. Burgen, rye, sourdough) ❋ ½ wholegrain bread roll ❋ ½ wholegrain flat bread ❋ 2 slices wholegrain or seeded crisp bread (e.g. Ryvita, Vita-Weat) ❋ ⅔ cup (30 g) high-fibre breakfast cereal flakes (those containing mixed or wholegrains such as buckwheat, puffed wheat or rice are good sources of resistant starch) ❋ ⅓ cup (30 g) uncooked rolled oats (⅔ cup cooked) ❋ ¼ cup (40 g) uncooked millet, barley or quinoa (¾ cup cooked) ❋ ½ cup (50 g) cooked wholemeal pasta ❋ ½ cup (75 g) cooked basmati rice, buckwheat, couscous, semolina, polenta ❋ ½ cup (100 g) baked beans or other cooked legumes ❋ 1 medium (150 g) potato or sweet potato ❋ 1 heaped tablespoon (30 g) pure maize corn flour, potato starch, chickpea flour, green banana flour, millet flour or rice flour
Lean meat, fish, poultry, eggs, tofu (3 units a day: 1 for lunch and 2 for dinner)	❋ 100 g (raw weight) lamb, beef, veal or kangaroo (maximum 500 g per week) ❋ 100 g (raw weight) fish and seafood (minimum twice-weekly) ❋ 100 g (raw weight) chicken, turkey, duck or pork ❋ 2 eggs (large) ❋ 1 cup (150 g) cooked or canned lentils, beans, chickpeas or other legumes (minimum twice-weekly) ❋ 170 g tofu or Quorn products
Fruit (2 units a day)	❋ 150 g fresh fruit (1 medium apple, 1 banana, 1 pear, 1 orange, 1 tangerine or 1 peach) ❋ 2 small fresh fruits (e.g. apricots, kiwi fruit, plums, nectarines, feijoas) ❋ 1 cup diced fresh, frozen or canned fruit (no juice) (e.g. berries, pineapple, mango, cherries, grapes)

PORTIONS/QUANTITIES PER UNIT

Food group	1 unit
Vegetables (a minimum of 5 units a day; see the 'Eat Freely' table overleaf)	• 1 cup (approx. 150 g) cooked vegetables • 2 cups (approx. 150 g) raw leafy green vegetables (e.g. lettuce, spinach, watercress, rocket) or raw salad vegetables (e.g. tomato, cucumber, beetroot, radish)
Dairy (3 units a day)	• 1 cup (250 ml) fresh, UHT, powdered or buttermilk • 1 cup (250 ml) calcium-fortified soy, almond or rice milk • ¾ cup (200 g) yoghurt • ½ cup (120 g) ricotta cheese • ½ cup (100 g) cottage cheese • 40 g cheddar or other full-fat cheese
Healthy fats and oils (4 units a day)	• 1 teaspoon (5 ml) olive oil, canola oil or sunflower oil • 1 teaspoon (5 g) margarine, rice bran oil or grapeseed oil • 1 tablespoon (20 g) avocado • 1 tablespoon (30 g) LSA (linseed, soy and almond meal) • 7 g nuts (e.g. 7 cashews, 7 almonds, 3 brazil nuts)
Indulgence foods (No more than 9 units per week as each is 450 kJ)	• 150 ml wine • 30 ml spirits • 375 ml beer • 20 g chocolate • 45 g (1 tablespoon) jam, honey, marmalade or maple syrup • 30 g (4–5) small pieces confectionery (lollies) • 20 g potato chips, corn chips or savoury 'snack' foods • 8 x deep-fried hot chips (fries) • 40 g (2 tablespoons) tomato, sweet chilli, plum or barbecue sauce • 1 small muesli bar • 2 small plain sweet biscuits (e.g. shortbread or milk arrowroot; check the packet as chocolate ones are much higher in energy) • 40 g slice of cake or sweet bun • 10–12 rice crackers

THE 'EAT-FREELY' FOODS

Vegetables		
Artichoke	Cauliflower	Onion
Asparagus	Celeriac	Parsnip
Bamboo shoots	Celery	Pumpkin
Beetroot	Choko	Radish
Bok choy and other Asian greens (e.g. choy sum, gai lan, water spinach)	Cucumber	Shallots
	Eggplant	Silverbeet
	Fennel	Snow peas
	Green beans	Spinach
Broccoli	Green peas	Spring onion
Brussels sprouts	Kale	Sprouts
Cabbages, all types, including red	Leek	Squash
	Lettuce (e.g. cos, mignonette)	Tomato
Capsicum		Turnip
Carrot	Mushrooms	Zucchini
Cassava	Okra	

Beverages

Herbal black teas, black coffee, unflavoured mineral or soda waters, water and naturally flavoured water (using fruit essences such as sliced citrus, cucumber, mint etc)

Herbs, spices and condiments		
Basil	Garlic	Soy sauce
Chicory	Ginger	Stock cubes
Chilli	Hoisin sauce	Turmeric
Chives	Lemon	Vinegar
Curry powder	Mint	Wasabi
Fish sauce	Parsley	

- Fresh and dried herbs along with whole and ground spices can be used freely

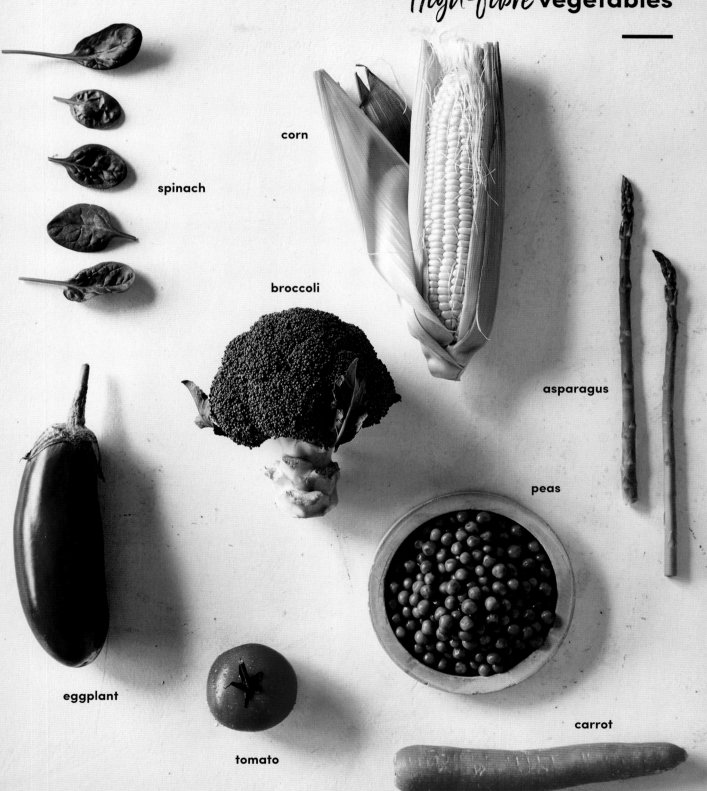

High-fibre **vegetables**

corn

spinach

broccoli

asparagus

peas

eggplant

carrot

tomato

How to use the *recipes* and sample *meal plans*

All the recipes in this book have been designed with fibre and gut health in mind.

Most contain higher amounts of fibre and resistant starch to feed the gut microbiota. The aim is to consume a minimum of 25 grams a day, from a range of sources. The fibre flag (see below) indicates the amount of fibre contained in the recipes. Use the fibre flags to ensure an adequate daily fibre intake.

Important note: If your diet is currently low in fibre, increase the fibre content gradually to allow your digestive system time to adapt, and don't forget to increase your water intake to maintain regularity.

For greater flexibility, combine a lower-fibre meal (3–5 g) with two high-fibre meals (<10 g) on the same day to balance things out, and if you have a busy schedule and don't have time to prepare snacks, have a banana or a handful of cashews to boost resistant starch, or simply increase your intake of high-fibre vegetables.

We have also provided several nutritionally complete sample days to demonstrate how you can use the daily food guide to reach your fibre target across the day, based on some common food preferences, including:

- a dairy-free day
- a low-FODMAP day
- a resistant starch day
- a wheat- and dairy-free day
- a wheat-free day.

What if I'm on a low-FODMAP diet?

We understand that some of our readers may already be progressing on a low-FODMAP diet (under the supervision of their healthcare team) for the management of their professionally diagnosed IBS symptoms. For this reason, we have taken the care to incorporate a low-FODMAP flag (see below) to guide the selection of suitable recipe choices. As each individual digests FODMAPs differently, we encourage you to discuss the use of these recipes with your team so you are getting the most from your diet.

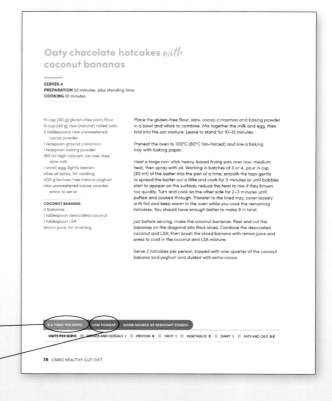

fibre flag

low-FODMAP flag

HIGH-FODMAP FOODS AND THEIR ALTERNATIVES

Food category	High-FODMAP foods	Low-FODMAP alternatives
Vegetables	Artichokes, asparagus, beetroot, broccoli, brussels sprouts, cauliflower, garlic, leek, onion, savoy cabbage, sugar snap peas, sweet corn	Alfalfa or bean sprouts, bok choy, carrot, celery, choy sum, cucumber, eggplant, green beans, lettuce, olives, parsnip, potato, pumpkin, spinach, sweet potato, tomato, zucchini
Fruit	Apple, blackberries, boysenberries, dried fruit, figs, mango, pear, prunes, stone fruit (nectarine, peach, plum), watermelon	Banana, blueberries, grapes, honeydew melon, kiwi fruit, mandarin, orange, passionfruit, pineapple, raspberries, strawberries
Dairy and dairy alternatives	Milk and yoghurt from cows/goats; soft cheese, cream	Lactose-free milk, ice cream and yoghurt; hard cheese, parmesan, camembert, feta, mozzarella
Meat and other protein sources	Chickpeas, beans, red and green lentils, tofu (silken, drained and firm, undrained)	All lean meats, fish, poultry, canned lentils, eggs, tofu (firm, drained only)
Breads and cereals	Rye, rolled oats (not instant oats); wheat-containing breads; wheat-based cereals, wheat pasta, wheat or rye cracker biscuits, sweet biscuits, cakes	Gluten-free bread, cakes and biscuits; sourdough spelt bread, rice bubbles, oats, gluten-free pasta, rice, quinoa
Nuts and seeds	Cashews, pistachios, almonds, hazelnuts	Macadamias, brazil nuts, peanuts, pecans, seeds
Beverages	Strong tea, ciders, sweet wines, chamomile tea	Weak tea, coffee, diet cordial, lemonade, dry wines, beer, peppermint tea
Miscellaneous	Margarine and butter containing lactose; onion and garlic salts; apricot jam; honey; ice cream; milk chocolate	Lactose-free spreads, fresh herbs, garlic-infused olive oil, peanut butter; dark chocolate

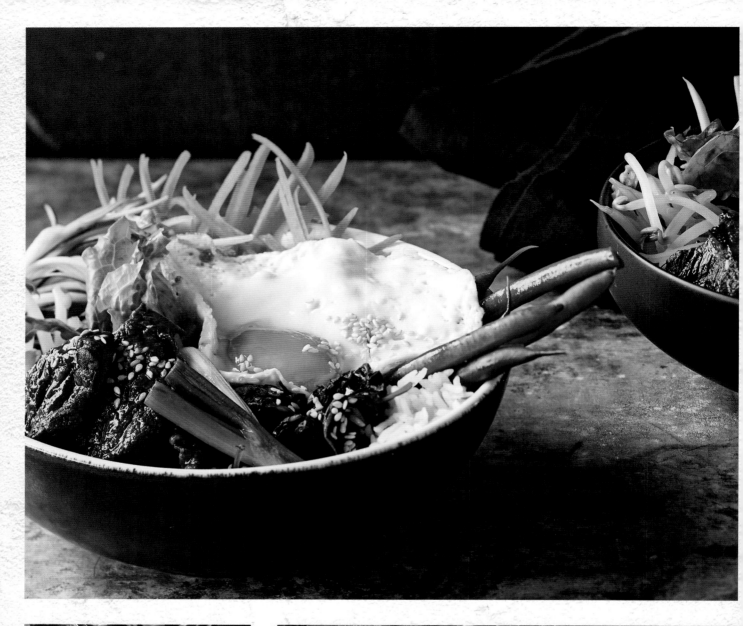

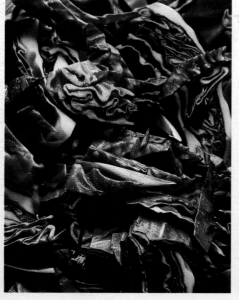

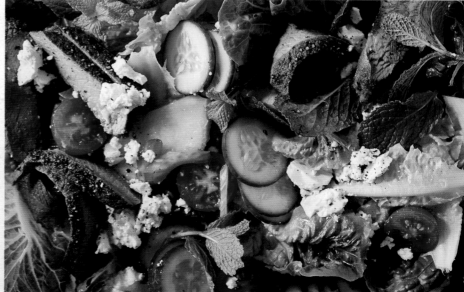

Daily *meal plan*: Dairy-free

Understanding that some of you may not be able to tolerate dairy in your daily diet, we have constructed a dairy-free day as an example to demonstrate how to use the foods in your diet to gain all the right nutrients, especially calcium.

Breakfast

Chai-spiced millet and brown rice porridge with orange and grapes (see page 72; swap the lactose-free milk for the same amount of calcium-fortified soy milk, and replace the lactose-free natural yoghurt with the same amount of soy yoghurt)

Units per serve:
- Breads and cereals **1**
- Fruit **0.5**
- Dairy **1** (alternative)
- Fats and oils **2**

Lunch

Sukiyaki beef bowl (see page 101)

Units per serve:
- Breads and cereals **1**
- Protein **1**
- Vegetables **2.5**

Dinner

Cheat's chicken paella (see page 138)

Units per serve:
- Breads and cereals **1**
- Protein **2**
- Vegetables **2**

Snacks

You can choose to have these snacks to top up between meals, or at mealtimes.

1 Cinnamon granola bar (see page 200):
- Breads and cereals **1**
- Fats and oils **1**

30 g soy cheese:
- Dairy **1**

7 cashews:
- Fats and oils **1**

75 g fresh fruit salad + 200 g soy yoghurt:
- Dairy **1**
- Fruit **½**

THIS DAILY MEAL PLAN PROVIDES 31 G FIBRE PER DAY

Daily *meal plan*: Low-FODMAP

Following the low-FODMAP diet can be helpful if you experience symptoms of IBS. This meal plan is suitable for the elimination phase of the low-FODMAP diet – but remember, the elimination phase isn't forever! The guide below will help you get the nutrients you need while you work towards reintroducing FODMAP foods into your diet. You will get the best results by doing this under the guidance of a dietitian.

Breakfast

Oaty chocolate hotcakes with coconut bananas (see page 68)

Units per serve:
- Breads and cereals **1**
- Fruit **1**
- Dairy (alternative) **1**
- Fats and oils **0.5**

Lunch

South-western prawn and green bean rice bowl (see page 100)

Units per serve:
- Breads and cereals **2**
- Protein **1**
- Vegetables **4**
- Dairy (alternative) **0.5**
- Fats and oils **1**

Dinner

Lamb, spinach, potato and pea curry with spiced rice (see page 172)

Units per serve:
- Breads and cereals **1**
- Protein **2**
- Vegetables **2**
- Fats and oils **0.5**

Snacks

You can choose to have these snacks to top up between meals, or at mealtimes.

Banana, berry and yoghurt smoothie (see page 199):
- Fruit **1**
- Dairy **1**

100 g lactose-free yoghurt:
- Dairy **0.5**

7 g cashews:
- Fats and oils **1**

THIS DAILY MEAL PLAN PROVIDES 30 G FIBRE PER DAY

Daily *meal plan*: High-fibre and resistant starch

When it comes to resistant starch, knowing which foods to include or how to prepare foods to improve your intake can be tricky. This sample meal plan shows you how easy it is to include good sources of resistant starch fibre. This plan is high in total fibre, so if you are starting from a low-fibre intake you may wish to speak to your health professional and introduce these options slowly.

Breakfast

Combine 75 g mashed banana, 125 ml reduced-fat milk and 40 g uncooked rolled oats. Top with 2 level teaspoons mixed seeds, 75 g mixed fresh or frozen berries and 100 g reduced-fat vanilla yoghurt.

Units per serve:
- Breads and cereals **1** * Fruit **1**
- Dairy (alternative) **1** * Fats and oils **2**

Lunch

Chunky barley, vegetable and chicken soup (see page 85)

Units per serve:
- Breads and cereals **2** * Protein **1**
- Vegetables **1.5**

Dinner

Pepper-crusted steaks with crushed peas and chargrilled vegetables (see page 165)

Units per serve:
- Breads and cereals **1** * Protein **2**
- Vegetables **2** * Dairy (alternative) **1**
- Fats and oils **1**

Snacks

You can choose to have these snacks to top up between meals, or at mealtimes.

150 g chopped watermelon: * Fruit **1**
1 small skim latte or 1 small tub (150 g) reduced-fat yoghurt or add 20 g parmesan to your lunch soup: * Dairy **1**

THIS DAILY MEAL PLAN PROVIDES 47 G FIBRE PER DAY

Daily *meal plan*: Wheat- and dairy-free

If you are unable to eat dairy or wheat, it is important to make sure you are still getting enough nutrients from alternative foods. Try calcium-fortified dairy alternatives like soy or almond milk, and use the guide below to increase fibre for good gut health.

Breakfast

Cinnamon, cashew and dried cranberry granola (see page 64; swap lactose-free milk for the same amount of a calcium-fortified non-dairy alternative)
Units per serve:
- Breads and cereals **1**
- Fruit **1**
- Dairy (alternative) **1**
- Fats and oils **1**

Lunch

Vietnamese chicken meatball and Asian slaw wraps (see page 95)

Units per serve:
- Breads and cereals **2**
- Protein **1**
- Vegetables **1**
- Fats and oils **0.5**

Dinner

Sumac-dusted prawns with quinoa 'tabbouleh' (see page 125)

Units per serve:
- Breads and cereals **1**
- Protein **2**
- Vegetables **2.5**
- Fats and oils **1**

Snacks

You can choose to have these snacks to top up between meals, or at mealtimes.

1 orange: Fruit **1**
250 ml almond or soy-milk latte: Dairy **1**
200 g soy yoghurt: Dairy (alternative) **1**
1 tablespoon Lemony nuts and olives (see page 215): Fats and oils **0.5**

THIS DAILY MEAL PLAN PROVIDES 30 G FIBRE PER DAY

Daily *meal plan*: Wheat-free

Wheat-based products usually come with valuable nutrients, as well as being a great source of fibre. If you are someone who experiences discomfort when eating wheat-based foods, it is important that you still get at least 25–30 g fibre each day. This plan will help you do that.

Breakfast

Lentil parathas with dhal, feta and kachumber salad (see page 77)

Units per serve:
- Breads and cereals **1** ❋ Protein **0.5**
- Vegetables **1.5** ❋ Dairy **1**

Lunch

Poached chicken waldorf sandwiches (see page 96; swap the bread for a wheat-free alternative such as Burgen Gluten Free)

Units per serve:
- Breads and cereals **2** ❋ Protein **1**
- Vegetables **0.5** ❋ Dairy (alternative) **0.5**
- Fats and oils **5**

Dinner

Bibimbap (see page 161)

Units per serve:
- Breads and cereals **1** ❋ Protein **2**
- Vegetables **2** ❋ Fats and oils **1.5**

Snacks

You can choose to have these snacks to top up between meals, or at mealtimes.

2 x 150 g pieces of fresh fruit: ❋ Fruit **2**
Add an extra 35 g cheese to your lunch sandwich or have 1 skim medium latte (375 ml): ❋ Dairy **1.5**
Add 25 g cheese to your lunch sandwich and have 100 g reduced-fat yoghurt: ❋ Dairy **1**

THIS DAILY MEAL PLAN PROVIDES 32 G FIBRE PER DAY

PART THREE

The Recipes

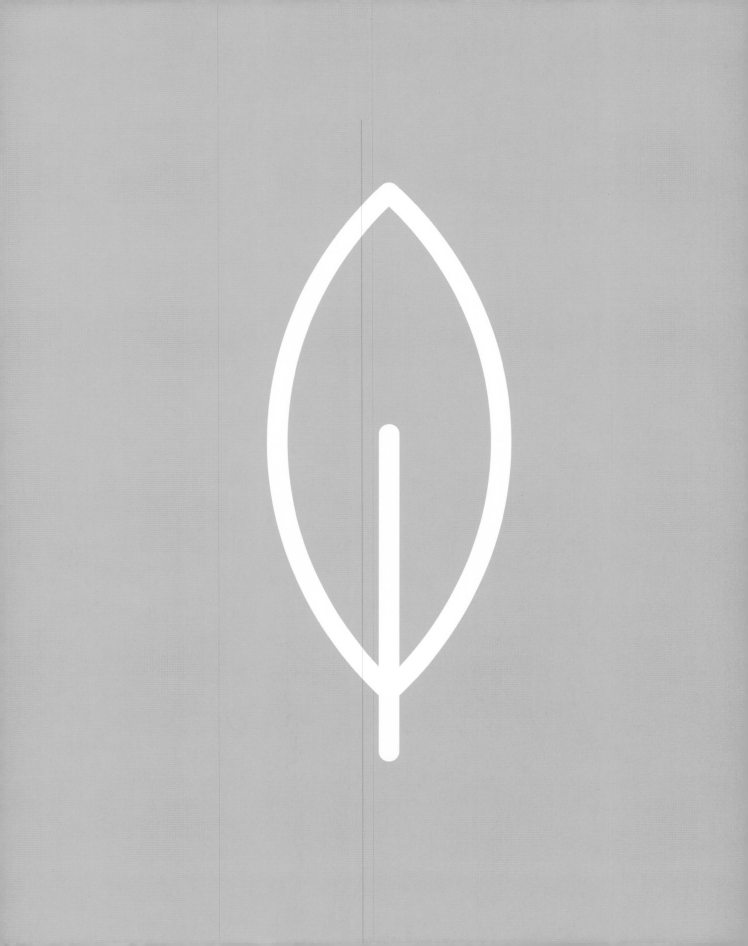

Breakfast

Cinnamon, cashew *and* dried cranberry granola

SERVES 4
PREPARATION 20 minutes
COOKING 35 minutes

1 litre high-calcium, lactose-free skim
  milk and 340 g pomegranate seeds,
  to serve

GRANOLA (Makes about 880 g = 29 serves)
4 cups (360 g) raw (natural) rolled oats
1½ cups (150 g) quinoa flakes
100 g raw cashews, roughly chopped
½ cup (70 g) raw almonds,
  roughly chopped
2 tablespoons LSA (or 1 tablespoon
  linseeds and 1 tablespoon
  sesame seeds)
3 teaspoons ground cinnamon
1 teaspoon ground ginger
½ cup (125 ml) boiling water
¼ cup (60 ml) pure maple syrup
1 teaspoon pure vanilla extract
140 g reduced-sugar dried cranberries

Preheat the oven to 140°C (120°C fan-forced). Line 2 large baking trays with baking paper.

Place the oats, quinoa flakes, cashews, almonds, LSA or seeds in a large bowl and stir to combine. Add the cinnamon and ginger and mix well.

Combine the boiling water, maple syrup and vanilla in a heatproof jug and pour over the oat mixture, then stir to mix it through evenly; the oat mixture should be slightly damp but not wet.

Divide the oat mixture between the trays, spreading it out to form an even layer.

Bake for 35 minutes until fragrant and golden. Leave to cool on the trays, then stir through the cranberries. Store in an airtight container for up to 3 weeks. Scoop one serve into each of 4 bowls and top with one-quarter of the skim milk and pomegranate seeds.

This recipe makes a large batch of granola which will keep in an airtight container for up to 3 weeks. For four people, serve ¼ cup (30 g) granola per person, with 1 cup (250 ml) high-calcium, lactose-free skim milk and 85 g pomegranate seeds per serve.

If you are sensitive to FODMAPS, swap cashews for low-FODMAP nuts (brazil/macadamia/pecan/hazelnuts); and reduce the serve of pomegranate seeds to 40 g per serve.

8 G FIBRE PER SERVE **GOOD SOURCE OF RESISTANT STARCH**

UNITS PER SERVE ❀ BREADS AND CEREALS **1** ❀ PROTEIN **0** ❀ FRUIT **1** ❀ VEGETABLES **0** ❀ DAIRY **1** ❀ FATS AND OILS **1**

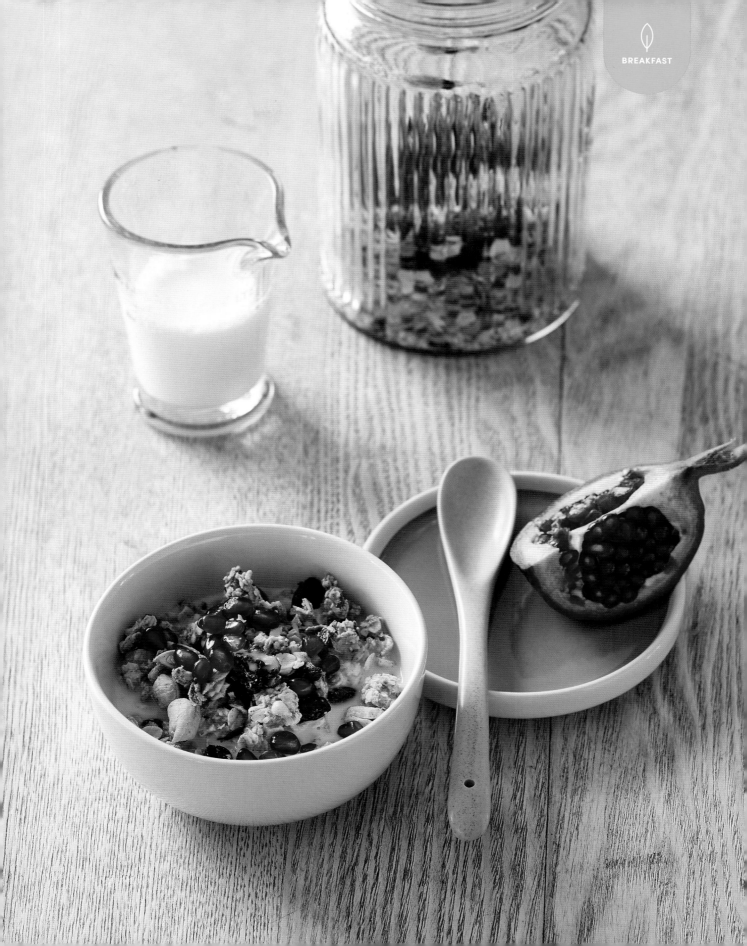

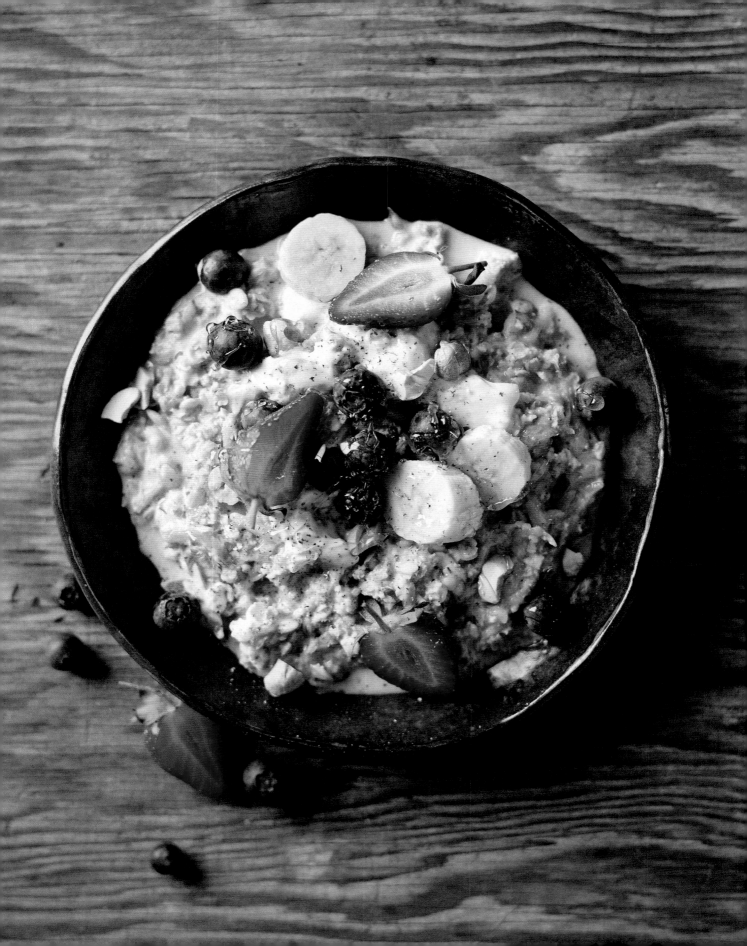

Bircher muesli *with* banana *and* berries

SERVES 4
PREPARATION 20 minutes, plus refrigerating time
COOKING Nil

Uncooked rolled oats have around three times the amount of resistant starch as cooked oats.

2 cups (180 g) raw (natural) rolled oats
¼ cup (20 g) brown rice flakes
juice of 2 oranges
⅓ cup (80 ml) boiling water,
  or as needed
freshly grated nutmeg, to taste
125 g blueberries
250 g strawberries, hulled and
  quartered or sliced
800 g lactose-free natural
  or vanilla yoghurt
2 teaspoons pure maple syrup
2 tablespoons raw cashews, roasted
1 small banana, sliced or diced

Combine the oats, brown rice flakes and orange juice in a bowl. Add enough boiling water to ensure the mixture is almost covered in liquid, then grate over a little nutmeg to taste. Cover with plastic film and refrigerate for a minimum of 2 hours or overnight, if time permits.

Just before serving, stir in the blueberries and half of the strawberries, the yoghurt and maple syrup.

Divide the bircher muesli among 4 bowls and top evenly with the cashews, banana and remaining strawberries. Serve with extra grated nutmeg, if desired.

If you are sensitive to FODMAPS, swap cashews for low-FODMAP nuts (brazil/macadamia/pecan/hazelnuts).

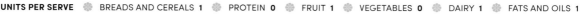

12 G FIBRE PER SERVE   GOOD SOURCE OF RESISTANT STARCH

UNITS PER SERVE ❀ BREADS AND CEREALS **1** ❀ PROTEIN **0** ❀ FRUIT **1** ❀ VEGETABLES **0** ❀ DAIRY **1** ❀ FATS AND OILS **1**

Oaty chocolate hotcakes *with* coconut bananas

SERVES 4
PREPARATION 20 minutes, plus standing time
COOKING 10 minutes

⅔ cup (100 g) gluten-free plain flour
½ cup (45 g) raw (natural) rolled oats
2 tablespoons raw unsweetened
    cocoa powder
1 teaspoon ground cinnamon
1 teaspoon baking powder
150 ml high-calcium, lactose-free
    skim milk
1 small egg, lightly beaten
olive oil spray, for cooking
400 g lactose-free natural yoghurt
raw unsweetened cocoa powder,
    extra, to serve

COCONUT BANANAS

4 bananas
1 tablespoon desiccated coconut
1 tablespoon LSA
lemon juice, for brushing

Place the gluten-free flour, oats, cocoa, cinnamon and baking powder in a bowl and whisk to combine. Mix together the milk and egg, then fold into the oat mixture. Leave to stand for 10–15 minutes.

Preheat the oven to 100°C (80°C fan-forced) and line a baking tray with baking paper.

Heat a large non-stick heavy-based frying pan over low–medium heat, then spray with oil. Working in batches of 3 or 4, pour ⅓ cup (80 ml) of the batter into the pan at a time, smooth the tops gently to spread the batter out a little and cook for 3 minutes or until bubbles start to appear on the surface; reduce the heat to low if they brown too quickly. Turn and cook on the other side for 2–3 minutes until puffed and cooked through. Transfer to the lined tray, cover loosely with foil and keep warm in the oven while you cook the remaining hotcakes. You should have enough batter to make 8 in total.

Just before serving, make the coconut bananas. Peel and cut the bananas into thick slices. Combine the desiccated coconut and LSA, then brush the sliced banana with lemon juice and press to coat in the coconut and LSA mixture.

Serve 2 hotcakes per person, topped with one-quarter of the coconut banana and yoghurt and dusted with extra cocoa.

8 G FIBRE PER SERVE | **LOW FODMAP** | **GOOD SOURCE OF RESISTANT STARCH**

UNITS PER SERVE BREADS AND CEREALS **1** PROTEIN **0** ❄ FRUIT **1** ❄ VEGETABLES **0** DAIRY **1** ❄ FATS AND OILS **0.5**

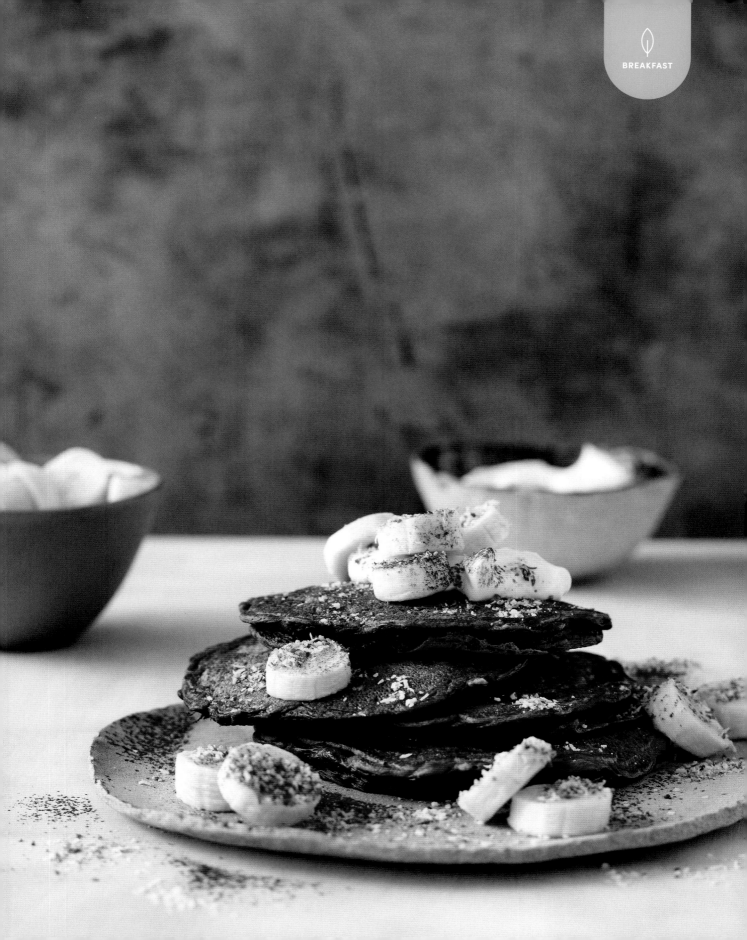

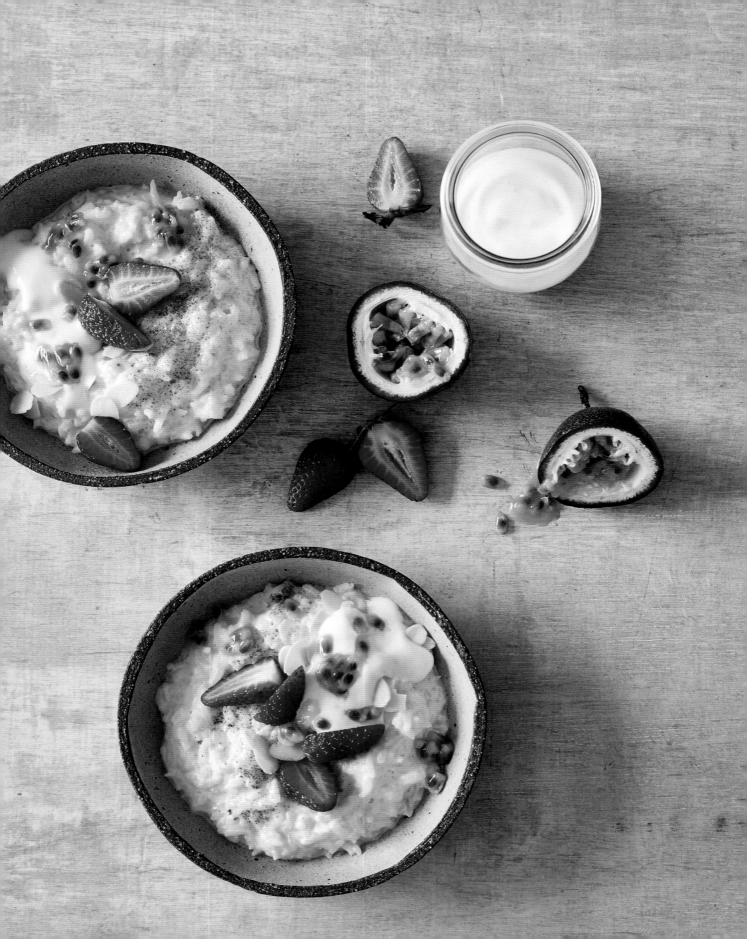

Brekky rice pudding *with* fruit *and* almonds

SERVES 4
PREPARATION 10 minutes
COOKING 25 minutes

½ cup (100 g) basmati rice
600 ml high-calcium, lactose-free
   skim milk
½ stick cinnamon
1 large wide strip lemon zest
1 teaspoon pure vanilla extract
2 teaspoons pure maple syrup
ground cinnamon, to serve
seeds and juice from 4 passionfruit
125 g strawberries, hulled and halved
   or quartered
20 g flaked almonds
2 tablespoons lactose-free natural
   yoghurt, to serve

Bring a small saucepan of water to the boil, then add the rice and boil for 5 minutes. Drain and transfer to a heavy-based saucepan. Add the milk, cinnamon, lemon zest and vanilla and bring to the boil over medium heat. Reduce the heat to low–medium and simmer, stirring frequently, for 20 minutes or until the milk is absorbed, the rice is cooked and the mixture is thick. Stir in the maple syrup.

Divide the rice pudding among 4 bowls, sprinkle with ground cinnamon to taste, then top evenly with the passionfruit, strawberries and almonds and serve warm with yoghurt.

This can be made the day before and chilled in the refrigerator overnight, if desired. The pudding will thicken on chilling, so loosen with a little extra skim milk, if you like.

7 G FIBRE PER SERVE   **LOW FODMAP**

UNITS PER SERVE   BREADS AND CEREALS **0.5**   PROTEIN **0**   FRUIT **1**   VEGETABLES **0**   DAIRY **1**   FATS AND OILS **1**

Chai-spiced millet *and* brown rice porridge *with* orange *and* grapes

SERVES 4
PREPARATION 15 minutes
COOKING 6 minutes

180 g millet flake and brown rice flake porridge

620 ml high-calcium, lactose-free skim milk

¼–½ teaspoon ground cinnamon

¼ teaspoon freshly grated nutmeg

⅛ teaspoon ground ginger

⅛ teaspoon ground cardamom

1 orange

½ cup seedless red grapes, quartered or sliced

200 g lactose-free natural yoghurt or 1 cup (250 ml) high-calcium, lactose-free skim milk

1 tablespoon pure maple syrup

50 g unsalted hazelnuts or pecans, roughly chopped

Place the porridge in a heavy-based saucepan, then add the milk, 620 ml water, cinnamon, nutmeg, ginger and cardamom and bring to a simmer over medium heat. Reduce the heat to low–medium and cook, stirring constantly, for 6 minutes or until thick and creamy.

Meanwhile, peel the orange, then, using a small, sharp knife, cut between the membrane to remove the segments.

Divide the porridge among 4 bowls. Top each bowl with one-quarter of the orange segments, grapes, yoghurt or skim milk and maple syrup, scatter evenly with the chopped nuts and serve.

7 G FIBRE PER SERVE   **LOW FODMAP**

UNITS PER SERVE ❀ BREADS AND CEREALS **1** ❀ PROTEIN **0** ❀ FRUIT **1** ❀ VEGETABLES **0** ❀ DAIRY **1** ❀ FATS AND OILS **2**

Breakfast tortillas

SERVES 4
PREPARATION 15 minutes
COOKING 15 minutes

Because of its protein unit, you may prefer to serve this dish for a weekend brunch rather than breakfast.

4 taco shells
2 eggs
¼ cup (60 ml) skim milk
½ teaspoon ground cumin
160 g reduced-fat cheddar,
    coarsely grated
80 g avocado, diced into 1 cm pieces
lime wedges and Tabasco Chipotle
    Pepper Sauce (available from larger
    supermarkets, optional), to serve

REFRIED BEANS

olive oil spray, for cooking
½ small red onion, finely chopped
½ small red capsicum, seeded and
    finely chopped
1 small clove garlic, finely chopped
2 teaspoons ground cumin
⅓ cup (80 ml) salt-reduced
    tomato passata
1 × 400 g tin salt-reduced kidney beans,
    drained and rinsed

To make the refried beans, heat a heavy-based saucepan or frying pan over medium heat and spray with olive oil. Add the onion and capsicum and cook for 5 minutes or until softened. Add the garlic and cumin and cook for 30 seconds or until fragrant; add 1 tablespoon water if necessary to prevent the ingredients from sticking. Pour in the passata and kidney beans and stir to mix well, then crush lightly with a vegetable masher. Bring to a simmer, then reduce the heat to low, cover and simmer for 5–6 minutes until reduced and thick. Season with freshly ground black pepper and set aside.

Meanwhile, preheat the oven to 180°C (160°C fan-forced). Place the taco shells on a baking tray and bake according to the packet instructions.

Break the eggs into a small bowl, add the milk and cumin and lightly whisk together. Heat a small non-stick heavy-based frying pan over medium heat. Pour in the egg mixture and cook, continuously dragging the egg towards the centre of the pan, tilting the pan so the uncooked egg runs to the side, until all the egg is cooked. Remove from the heat. Either add the grated cheese to the scrambled egg or scatter it in the taco shells before serving.

Place the taco shells on a chopping board and divide half of the refried beans among them. Top with one-quarter of the scrambled egg and cheese, then finish with the avocado. Serve with lime wedges and Tabasco sauce, if desired.

You will only need to use half the refried beans here. The leftovers can be stored in an airtight container in the refrigerator or frozen for up to 1 month and used with the Fish tacos on page 129 or for Breakfast tortillas another day. Alternatively, halve the recipe to make half the amount.

5 G FIBRE PER SERVE | **GOOD SOURCE OF RESISTANT STARCH**

UNITS PER SERVE ❋ BREADS AND CEREALS **1.5** ❋ PROTEIN **1** ❋ FRUIT **0** ❋ VEGETABLES **0** ❋ DAIRY **1** ❋ FATS AND OILS **1**

Brekky fritters *with* smoked salmon *and* herbed goat's cheese

SERVES 4 (Makes 8 cakes)
PREPARATION 20 minutes
COOKING 15 minutes, plus potato cooking time

8 thin slices (400 g) smoked salmon

HERBED GOAT'S CHEESE
115 g soft goat's cheese (such as
    a small log of Bourdin chevre)
2 tablespoons finely chopped chives
2 tablespoons finely chopped
    flat-leaf parsley leaves

BREKKY FRITTERS
¾ cup (90 g) frozen peas
500 g potatoes, quartered, steamed
    and chilled overnight (see page 41)
1½ tablespoons skim milk
1 tablespoon light sour cream
150 g cabbage, thinly sliced
2 spring onions, finely chopped
2 tablespoons plain flour,
    plus extra for dusting
olive oil spray, for cooking

To make the herbed goat's cheese, place the cheese, chives and parsley in a small bowl and stir to combine well. Cover with plastic film and refrigerate until required.

To make the fritters, cook the peas in a small saucepan of boiling water for 5 minutes or until tender, then drain and set aside. Place the cooked potato in a large bowl and roughly mash with a vegetable masher. Add the milk and sour cream and roughly mash. Add the peas, cabbage and spring onion and stir to combine, then fold in the flour. Divide the mixture into 8 even portions and, using lightly floured hands, form into patties.

Heat a large non-stick heavy-based frying pan over medium heat, then spray with olive oil. Dust both sides of each patty lightly with flour, then place in the pan and cook over low–medium heat for 3–4 minutes on each side or until golden. (Depending on the size of your pan you may need to do this in batches.)

Serve the fritters warm with smoked salmon and herbed goat's cheese.

5 G FIBRE PER SERVE   **GOOD SOURCE OF RESISTANT STARCH**

UNITS PER SERVE ✦ BREADS AND CEREALS **2** ✦ PROTEIN **1** ✦ FRUIT **0** ✦ VEGETABLES **1** ✦ DAIRY **1.5** ✦ FATS AND OILS **1**

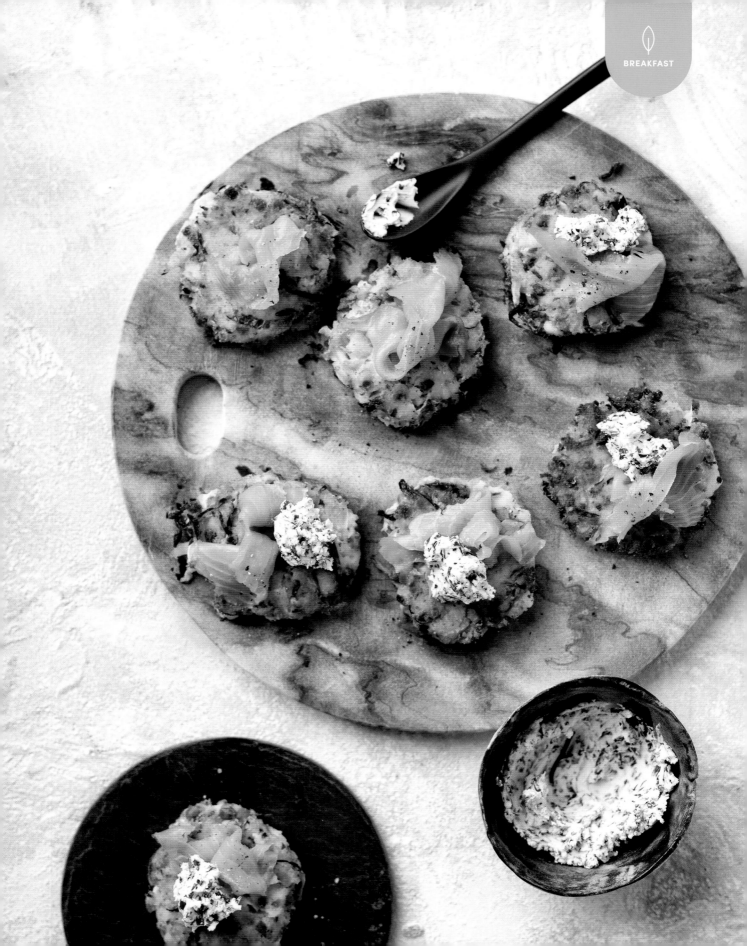

Lebanese breakfast plate

SERVES 4
PREPARATION 20 minutes
COOKING 15 minutes

Due to the protein and breads and cereals units in this dish, it is best enjoyed for brunch rather than breakfast.

4 eggs
1 quantity Spice-roasted
    Chickpeas (see page 208)
2 Lebanese cucumbers,
    quartered lengthways
2 roma tomatoes,
    quartered lengthways
4 wholemeal pita breads

SMASHED BROAD BEAN,
FETA AND MINT DIP
(MAKES ABOUT 2 CUPS/540 G)
500 g frozen broad beans
1 small clove garlic, crushed
1 tablespoon tahini
150 g salt-reduced feta
1 tablespoon reduced-fat natural
    Greek-style yoghurt
3 teaspoons lemon juice, or to taste
2 tablespoons roughly
    chopped mint leaves

To make the broad bean dip, cook the broad beans in a large saucepan of simmering water for 3 minutes, then drain, run under cold water and double-peel. Transfer to a blender or food processor and add the garlic, tahini and feta and blend or pulse until almost smooth. Add the yoghurt and lemon juice and blend or pulse until smooth. Season to taste with freshly ground black pepper, then stir in the mint. Taste and add extra lemon juice, if desired.

Boil the eggs in a saucepan of simmering water for 7 minutes for medium–hard-boiled or cook for another 2–3 minutes for hard-boiled. Drain, run under cold water, then peel and cut in half or into quarters.

Divide half of the broad bean dip among 4 long plates, add one-quarter of the spiced chickpeas, one-quarter of the cucumber and tomatoes, a boiled egg and a wholemeal pita bread to each plate, then serve. Store the remaining broad bean dip in an airtight container in the refrigerator for up to 4 days.

To adapt this to serve at breakfast, omit the wholemeal pita bread to reduce the breads and cereals units to 1, and omit the eggs to reduce the protein units.

The smashed broad bean dip makes twice as much as you need – use the leftovers in the Lamb wraps on page 92 or serve as a snack with crudites, such as carrot sticks, celery sticks, raw capsicum strips, snow peas, radishes or witlof leaves.

11 G FIBRE PER SERVE   **GOOD SOURCE OF RESISTANT STARCH**

UNITS PER SERVE   BREADS AND CEREALS **2**   PROTEIN **1**   FRUIT **0**   VEGETABLES **1**   DAIRY **1**   FATS AND OILS **1**

Lentil parathas *with* dhal, feta *and* kachumber salad

SERVES 4
PREPARATION 25 minutes, plus soaking time
COOKING 35 minutes

40 g Dhal (see page 211)
200 g salt-reduced low-fat feta,
    cut into bite-sized pieces
lemon wedges, to serve

LENTIL PARATHAS
25 g red lentils, soaked in cold
    water for 30 minutes
1 cup (150 g) gluten-free plain flour,
    plus extra for dusting
olive oil spray, for cooking

KACHUMBER SALAD
1 Lebanese cucumber, halved
    lengthways, then thinly sliced
    on the diagonal
2 roma tomatoes, halved and cut
    into thin wedges
2 teaspoons thinly sliced spring onion
    (green tops only)
1 teaspoon lime juice, or to taste
1 tablespoon coriander leaves

To make the parathas, drain and rinse the lentils, then place in a small blender or small food processor and process until a coarse puree forms. Transfer to a bowl, then gradually whisk in the flour, adding enough water to make a smooth dough (about ¼ cup/60 ml). Knead the dough gently to form a smooth ball.

Divide the dough into 4 even pieces and roll each one into a ball. Lightly dust a clean workbench with extra flour, then, using a lightly dusted rolling pin, roll the dough balls out until 1 mm thick.

Heat a non-stick heavy-based frying pan over medium heat and spray lightly with olive oil. Cook one dough round at a time, spraying the pan with extra oil as necessary to prevent sticking, for 3–4 minutes on each side until dry and golden brown bubbles appear. Transfer to a plate, cover with a clean tea towel and keep warm.

To make the kachumber salad, combine all the ingredients in a bowl.

Serve the parathas with the kachumber salad, dhal and feta, with lemon wedges on the side.

7 G FIBRE PER SERVE   **GOOD SOURCE OF RESISTANT STARCH**

UNITS PER SERVE   BREADS AND CEREALS **1**   PROTEIN **0.5**   FRUIT **0**   VEGETABLES **1.5**   DAIRY **1**   FATS AND OILS **0**

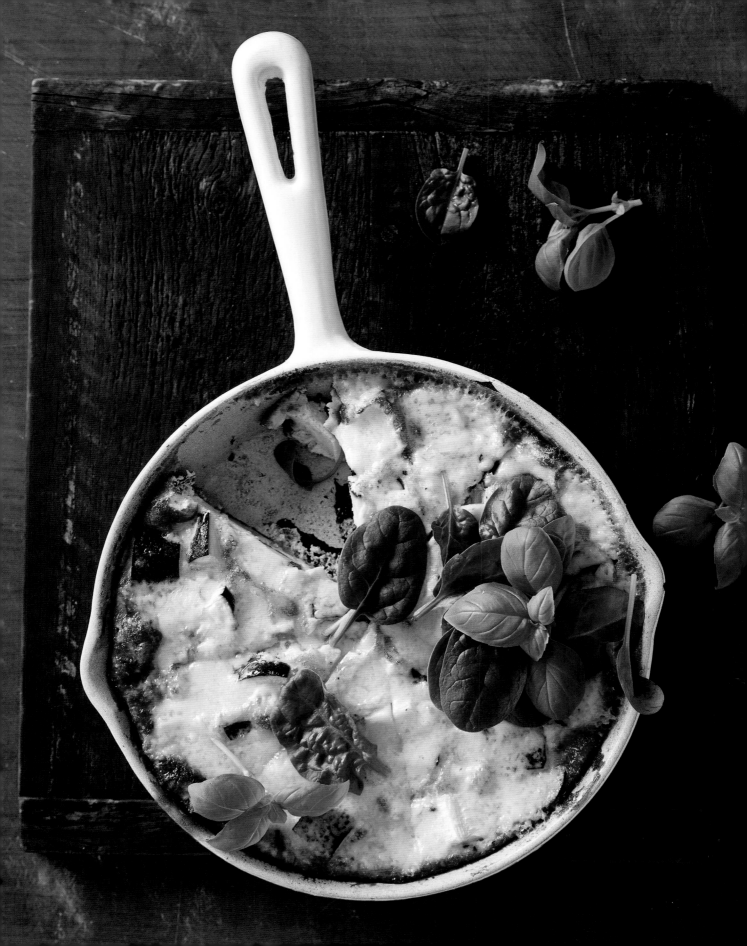

Zucchini frying-pan frittata

SERVES 4
PREPARATION 10 minutes
COOKING 15 minutes, plus resting time

When using this recipe, remember to reduce your portion of lean meat, fish, chicken or eggs at lunch or dinner by ½ unit.

1 tablespoon garlic-infused olive oil
2 zucchini, cut into 2 cm dice
1 stick celery, thinly sliced
½ cup (125 ml) lactose-free milk
4 eggs
100 g aged cheddar, crumbled
1 cup baby spinach leaves, trimmed
½ cup small basil leaves
4 slices gluten-free chia and sunflower
    bread, toasted

Heat the olive oil in a frying pan over medium heat. Add the zucchini and celery and cook, stirring, for 5 minutes or until softened and light golden.

Meanwhile, whisk together the milk and eggs in a jug and season with freshly ground black pepper.

Reduce the heat to low and pour the egg mixture into the pan. Stir gently for 20 seconds, then leave to cook, untouched, for 8 minutes or until the edges have set firm and the top and centre are still runny.

Preheat the oven grill to high.

Sprinkle the cheddar over the egg mixture, then place the pan under the grill for 2–3 minutes or until the cheese is melted and golden and the centre is completely set when tested with a knife.

Stand for 5 minutes, then cut into quarters and scatter with the combined spinach and basil. Serve each portion with a piece of toast alongside.

You can add 2 cups (270 g) chopped unpeeled sweet potato to the zucchini mixture in the pan – just cook it for an additional 5 minutes to soften. This will add 1 unit of breads and cereals per serve.

Celery is low-FODMAP in small quantities (up to ½ stick) – more than this is high-FODMAP.

4 G FIBRE PER SERVE   **LOW FODMAP**

UNITS PER SERVE ❋ BREADS AND CEREALS **1** ❋ PROTEIN **0.5** ❋ FRUIT **0** ❋ VEGETABLES **1.5** ❋ DAIRY **1** ❋ FATS AND OILS **1**

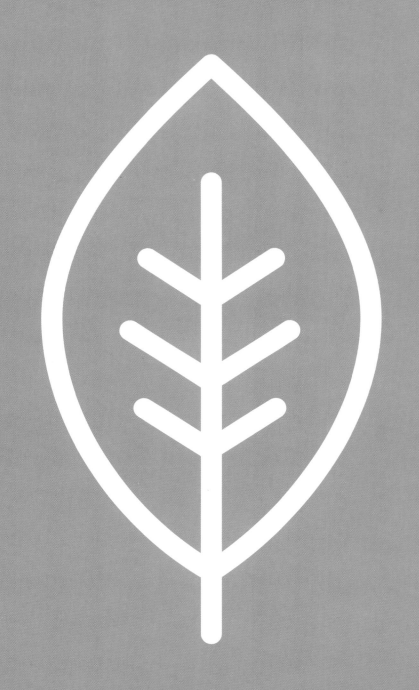

Lunch

Greek bean soup *with* crumbled feta

SERVES 4
PREPARATION 15 minutes
COOKING 2 hours 15 minutes

200 g dried cannellini beans
1 × 400 g tin salt-reduced
    chopped tomatoes
2 sticks celery, halved lengthways
    and cut into 1.5 cm thick slices,
    leafy tops reserved
3 small carrots, halved lengthways
    and cut into 1.5 cm thick slices
1 red onion, finely chopped
1½ teaspoons dried
    Greek-style oregano
pinch chilli powder (optional)
1 clove garlic, crushed
1 tablespoon extra virgin olive oil
¾ cup (165 g) small pasta such
    as risoni or orzo
200 g salt-reduced feta

Place the beans in a large heavy-based saucepan or stockpot, then cover with 3 litres water and bring to the boil over high heat. Reduce the heat to low–medium and simmer for 1 hour or until all the beans have sunk to the bottom of the pan. Drain, discarding the water, then return the beans to the pan.

Add the tomatoes, celery, celery tops, carrot, onion, 1 teaspoon of the oregano and chilli, if using. Cover with 2 litres cold water and bring to the boil over high heat. Reduce the heat to low–medium and simmer for 1 hour or until the beans are tender.

Using a mortar and pestle, crush the garlic with the remaining oregano leaves, then stir into the soup. Stir in the olive oil and season to taste with freshly ground black pepper. Add the pasta and cook for another 15 minutes or until it is al dente.

Ladle the soup into 4 bowls, then crumble 50 g feta over the top of each one and serve.

The beans don't need to be soaked in water before cooking in this recipe; it might sound odd, but it works!

17 G FIBRE PER SERVE   **GOOD SOURCE OF RESISTANT STARCH**

UNITS PER SERVE ❋ BREADS AND CEREALS **1** ❋ PROTEIN **1** ❋ FRUIT **0** ❋ VEGETABLES **2** ❋ DAIRY **1** ❋ FATS AND OILS **1**

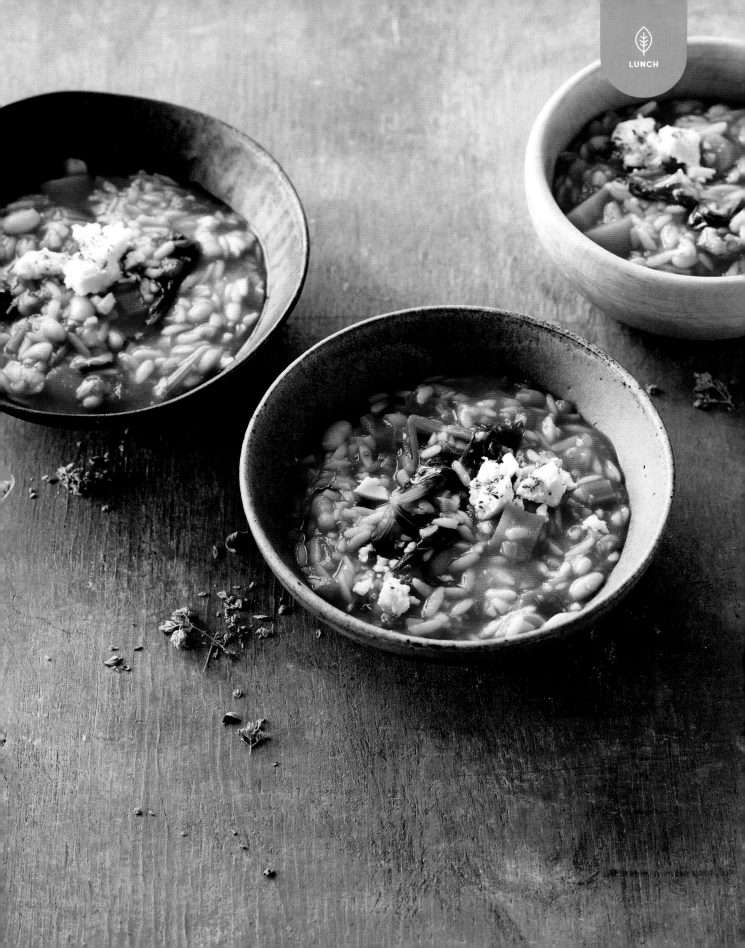

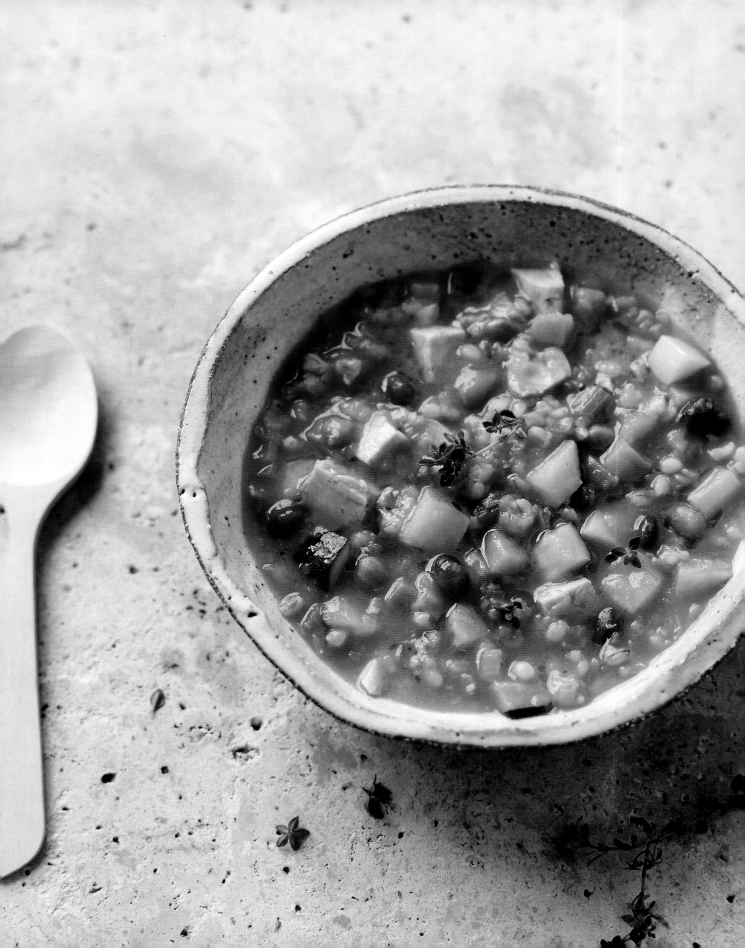

Chunky barley, vegetable *and* chicken soup

SERVES 4
PREPARATION 20 minutes
COOKING 2 hours, plus potato and sweet potato cooking time

olive oil spray, for cooking

2 leeks, white part only, finely chopped

2 carrots, finely chopped

3 sticks celery, cut into thirds lengthways and thinly sliced

2 tablespoons salt-reduced tomato paste

¾ cup (150 g) pearl barley, soaked in boiling water for 15 minutes

2 sprigs thyme (optional)

2 litres salt-reduced chicken or vegetable stock

2 desiree potatoes, cut into 1.5 cm dice, steamed and chilled overnight (see page 41)

1 small sweet potato (about 400 g), cut into 1.5 cm dice, steamed and chilled overnight (see page 41)

275 g chicken breast fillet

1 × 125 g tin salt-reduced four-bean mix, drained and rinsed

1 zucchini, cut into 1.5 cm dice

Heat a large heavy-based saucepan or stockpot over medium heat and spray with olive oil. Add the leek, carrot and celery and cook for 5 minutes or until softened but not coloured. Stir in the tomato paste to coat the vegetables. Drain the barley, then add to the pan with the thyme (if using) and stir to combine. Pour in 1.5 litres of the stock and bring to the boil over high heat. Cover, then reduce the heat to low and simmer for 45 minutes.

Add the potato and sweet potato and another 1 cup (250 ml) of the stock, then return to the boil. Reduce the heat to low, cover and cook for 45 minutes, then add the chicken and remaining stock to the pan and return to the boil. Reduce the heat to low and simmer, covered, for a further 20 minutes or until the chicken is cooked through. Remove the chicken from the pan and either cut into bite-sized pieces or shred with 2 forks.

Return the chicken to the pan, along with the beans and zucchini, and cook for 5 minutes or until heated through. Remove and discard the thyme. Ladle the soup evenly into 4 bowls and serve.

To save time, soak the barley in the boiling water while you prepare the vegetables.

18 G FIBRE PER SERVE   **GOOD SOURCE OF RESISTANT STARCH**

UNITS PER SERVE   BREADS AND CEREALS **2**   PROTEIN **1**   FRUIT **0**   VEGETABLES **1.5**   DAIRY **0**   FATS AND OILS **0**

Spiced pumpkin *and* chickpea soup *with* oat *and* parsley dumplings

---

SERVES 4–6
PREPARATION 25 minutes
COOKING 50 minutes

---

2 sticks celery, finely chopped
1 carrot, finely chopped
2 cm piece ginger, finely grated
2 teaspoons ground cumin
1 teaspoon ground coriander
½ teaspoon ground ginger
pinch of ground cinnamon
1 kg Kent or butternut pumpkin, peeled,
    seeded and roughly chopped
1 × 400 g tin salt-reduced chickpeas,
    drained and rinsed
2 teaspoons tahini, or to taste
chopped flat-leaf parsley leaves,
    to serve (optional)

OAT AND PARSLEY DUMPLINGS

1 cup (150 g) gluten-free
    self-raising flour
30 g salt-reduced vegan
    margarine spread, chopped
⅓ cup (30 g) raw (natural) rolled oats
2 tablespoons finely chopped
    flat-leaf parsley leaves
70 ml calcium-enriched almond milk

Heat a large heavy-based saucepan over medium heat and spray with olive oil. Add the celery and carrot and cook for 3 minutes or until soft but not coloured. Add the grated ginger and stir for 30 seconds, then add the cumin, coriander, ground ginger and cinnamon and stir for another 30 seconds or until fragrant. Add the pumpkin to the pan and stir to coat with the celery mixture, then pour in 3 cups (750 ml) water and bring to the boil. Add the chickpeas and stir, then reduce the heat to low–medium and simmer for 25 minutes or until the pumpkin is tender. Stir in the tahini.

Using a stick blender, blend the soup until a smooth puree forms.

Meanwhile, to make the dumplings, place the flour in a bowl, then rub in the margarine until a crumbly mixture forms. Stir in the oats and parsley, then slowly add the milk, stirring until a dough forms.

Pinch off small pieces of the dough, then, using lightly floured hands, roll into 1.5 cm diameter balls; you should have about 12. Place the dough balls on top of the soup – they will sink, but then float to the surface when they are cooked. Cover and cook over low heat for 15–20 minutes or until the dumplings are puffed and cooked through (test with a skewer – it should come out clean).

Divide the soup and dumplings among bowls, scatter with extra parsley, if desired, then serve.

---

12 G FIBRE PER SERVE   **GOOD SOURCE OF RESISTANT STARCH**

UNITS PER SERVE ✺ BREADS AND CEREALS **2** ✺ PROTEIN **1** ✺ FRUIT **0** ✺ VEGETABLES **3** ✺ DAIRY **0** ✺ FATS AND OILS **2**

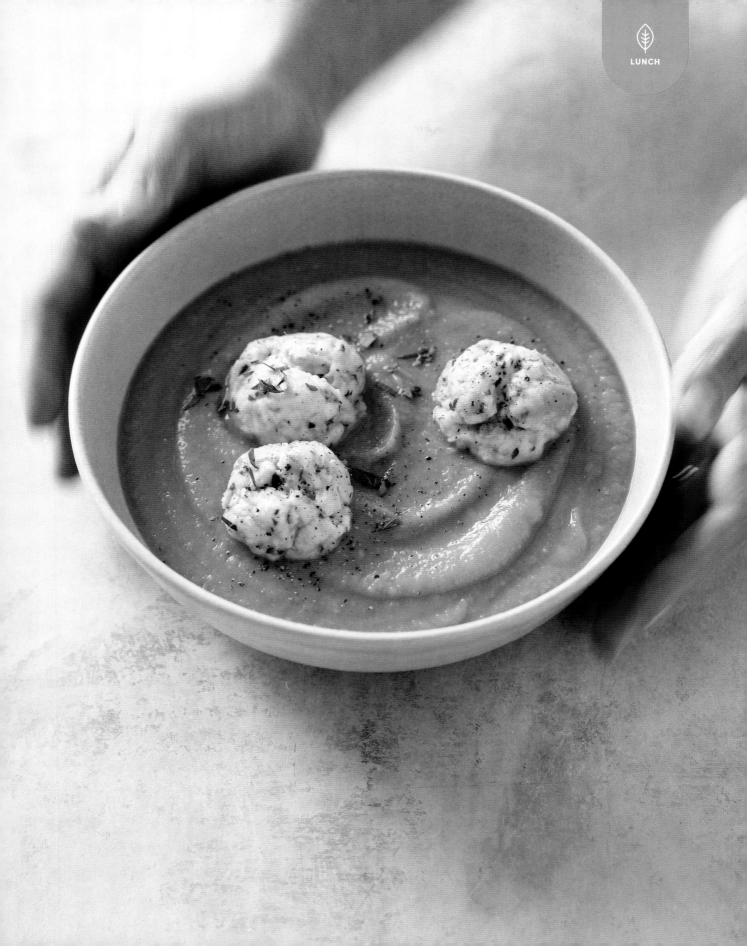

Indian-style lentil soup *with* spinach *and* lemon

SERVES 4
PREPARATION 20 minutes
COOKING 45 minutes, plus sweet potato cooking time

2 teaspoons olive oil
1 onion, finely chopped
1 carrot, finely chopped
1 stick celery, finely chopped
2 teaspoons curry powder
1 teaspoon ground cumin
1 teaspoon garam masala
¾ cup (150 g) brown lentils,
    rinsed and drained
½ cup (100 g) red lentils
1 × 400 g tin salt-reduced
    chopped tomatoes
1.25 litres salt-reduced chicken
    or vegetable stock
2 cups (240 g) frozen peas
1 small sweet potato (about 400 g),
    cut into 1.5 cm dice, steamed and
    chilled overnight (see page 41)
50 g poached shredded chicken
2 cups (150 g) baby spinach leaves,
    stems trimmed, shredded
lemon juice, to taste
4 wholemeal chapatis

Heat the olive oil in a heavy-based saucepan over medium–high heat, then add the onion, carrot and celery and cook, stirring, for 5–6 minutes or until softened. Add the curry powder, cumin and garam masala and stir for 1–2 minutes, until fragrant. Add the lentils, tomatoes and stock and stir to mix well. Bring to the boil, then reduce the heat to low and simmer for 25–30 minutes until the lentils are tender. Add the peas and sweet potato and cook for 3 minutes or until heated through, then remove from the heat. Mash coarsely with a potato masher, if desired.

Add the shredded chicken, spinach and lemon juice to taste, then stir just to heat through. Divide among 4 bowls and serve with the chapatis.

21 G FIBRE PER SERVE   GOOD SOURCE OF RESISTANT STARCH

UNITS PER SERVE ❋ BREADS AND CEREALS **2** ❋ PROTEIN **1** ❋ FRUIT **0** ❋ VEGETABLES **2** ❋ DAIRY **0** ❋ FATS AND OILS **0.5**

Brown rice, capsicum, currant *and* cashew salad

SERVES 4
PREPARATION 15 minutes, plus cooling time
COOKING 35 minutes

¾ cup (150 g) brown rice
⅓ cup (50 g) currants
boiling water, for soaking
1 red capsicum, seeded and finely diced
6 spring onions, finely chopped
20 g raw cashews, roasted
20 g sunflower seeds
1 tablespoon pumpkin seeds (pepitas)
1 tablespoon extra virgin olive oil
2 tablespoons salt-reduced soy sauce
1 tablespoon lemon juice
1 small clove garlic, crushed

Place the rice and 1½ cups (375 ml) water in a heavy-based saucepan and bring to the boil over high heat. Cover and reduce the heat to low, then cook for 35 minutes or until all the water has been absorbed and the rice is tender. Spread out on a baking tray and leave to cool.

Meanwhile, soak the currants in a small bowl of boiling water for 10 minutes, then drain and set aside.

Transfer the cooled rice to a large bowl, then add the currants, capsicum, spring onion, cashews, sunflower seeds and pumpkin seeds and stir to combine.

Place the olive oil, soy sauce, lemon juice and garlic in a bowl and stir to mix well.

Add the dressing to the salad and stir to mix through. Serve.

5 G FIBRE PER SERVE   **GOOD SOURCE OF RESISTANT STARCH**

UNITS PER SERVE   ❋ BREADS AND CEREALS **2**   ❋ PROTEIN **0**   ❋ FRUIT **0.5**   ❋ VEGETABLES **0.5**   ❋ DAIRY **0**   ❋ FATS AND OILS **2**

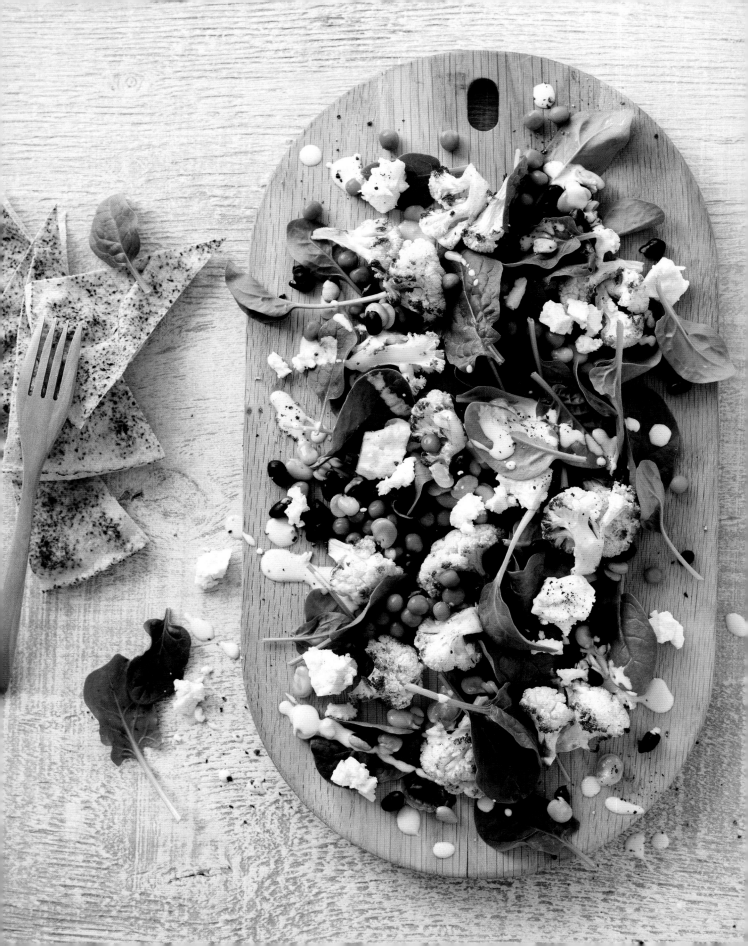

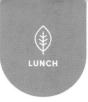
Cumin-roasted cauliflower *and* black bean salad *with* tahini dressing

SERVES 4
PREPARATION 20 minutes
COOKING 30 minutes

1 small or ½ large cauliflower,
    trimmed and cut into small florets
½ teaspoon ground cumin
olive oil spray, for cooking
200 g frozen broad beans
½ cup (60 g) frozen peas
200 g tinned salt-reduced
    black beans or cannellini beans,
    drained and rinsed
200 g baby spinach leaves,
    stems trimmed
180 g salt-reduced low-fat feta,
    crumbled or cut into small dice
2 wholemeal pita breads,
    cut into wedges

TAHINI DRESSING
1 small clove garlic, finely chopped
1 tablespoon tahini
1 tablespoon seasoned rice vinegar
½ teaspoon lemon juice, or to taste
1½ tablespoons boiling water,
    plus extra if needed
2 drops sesame oil

Preheat the oven to 200°C (180°C fan-forced) and line a baking tray with baking paper.

Place the cauliflower on the lined tray in a single layer, sprinkle with the ground cumin, then spray with olive oil. Roast, turning occasionally, for 30 minutes or until golden brown.

Meanwhile, cook the broad beans in a heavy-based saucepan of simmering water for 3 minutes or until tender, then drain and cool under cold running water. Double-peel, then place in a large bowl.

Cook the peas in a small heavy-based saucepan of simmering water for 3 minutes or until tender, then drain, cool under cold running water and add to the bowl with the broad beans. Add the black or cannellini beans and spinach to the bowl and gently stir to mix.

To make the tahini dressing, place the garlic, tahini, vinegar, lemon juice and boiling water in a small bowl and stir until smooth and well combined; add a little extra boiling water if necessary. Stir in the sesame oil and thin with a little more boiling water if a thinner consistency is desired.

Divide the broad bean mixture among 4 plates or bowls, then top evenly with the cauliflower and feta. Drizzle over the tahini dressing and serve with the pita wedges.

If preferred, you could use either 1 x 400 g tin of the salt-reduced beans, or 400 g of broad beans, as either of these makes up 1 protein unit.

14 G FIBRE PER SERVE | **GOOD SOURCE OF RESISTANT STARCH**

UNITS PER SERVE ✤ BREADS AND CEREALS **2** ✤ PROTEIN **1** ✤ FRUIT **0** ✤ VEGETABLES **1** ✤ DAIRY **1** ✤ FATS AND OILS **2**

Paprika lamb wraps *with* broad bean, feta *and* mint dip

SERVES 4
PREPARATION 15 minutes, plus resting time
COOKING 10 minutes

350 g lamb backstrap, all visible
    fat removed
½ teaspoon sweet paprika
½ teaspoon hot paprika
olive oil spray, for cooking
squeeze of lemon juice
4 gluten-free or rice wraps
⅓ cup (90 g) Smashed Broad Bean,
    Feta and Mint Dip (see page 76)
1 cup rocket leaves
1 tablespoon roughly chopped
    flat-leaf parsley or mint leaves
1 Lebanese cucumber, shaved
4 roma tomatoes, thinly sliced

Pat the lamb dry with paper towel, then sprinkle with both types of paprika and season with freshly ground black pepper, rubbing them in to coat the lamb evenly.

Heat a chargrill pan or heavy-based frying pan over medium–high heat, then spray the lamb with olive oil. Cook for 2–3 minutes on each side for medium–rare or continue until cooked to your liking. Cover loosely with foil and leave to rest for 5 minutes, then cut into slices and squeeze with lemon juice.

Spread each wrap with one-quarter of the broad bean dip, then top with one-quarter of the lamb, rocket, parsley or mint, cucumber and tomato. Roll up to enclose the filling and serve immediately.

5 G FIBRE PER SERVE

UNITS PER SERVE ❀ BREADS AND CEREALS **2** ❀ PROTEIN **1** ❀ FRUIT **0** ❀ VEGETABLES **1** ❀ DAIRY **0.5** ❀ FATS AND OILS **0**

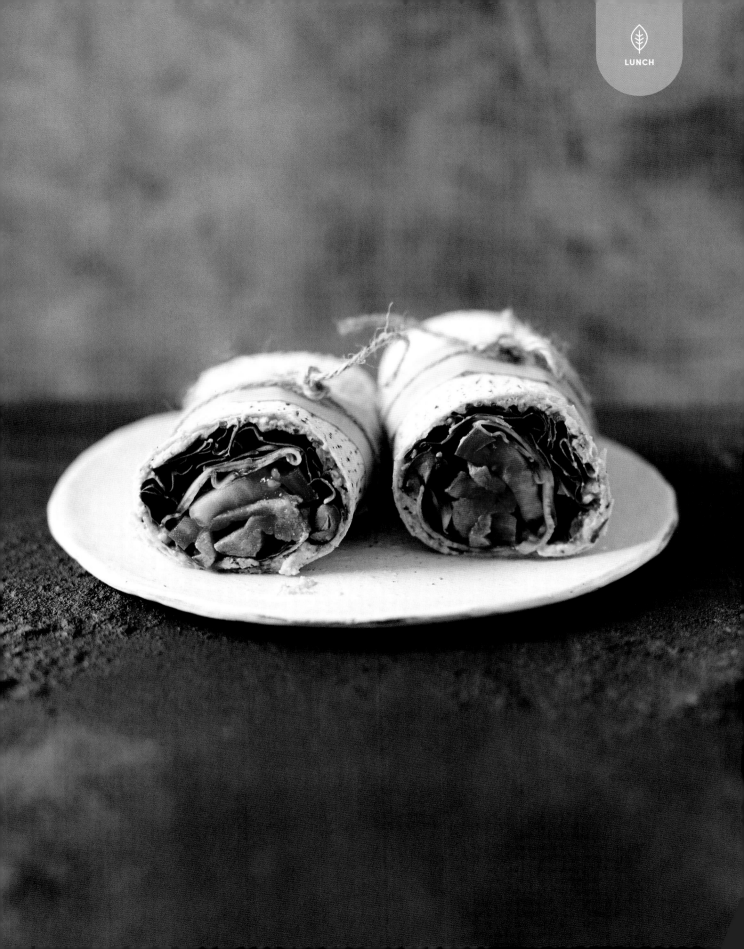

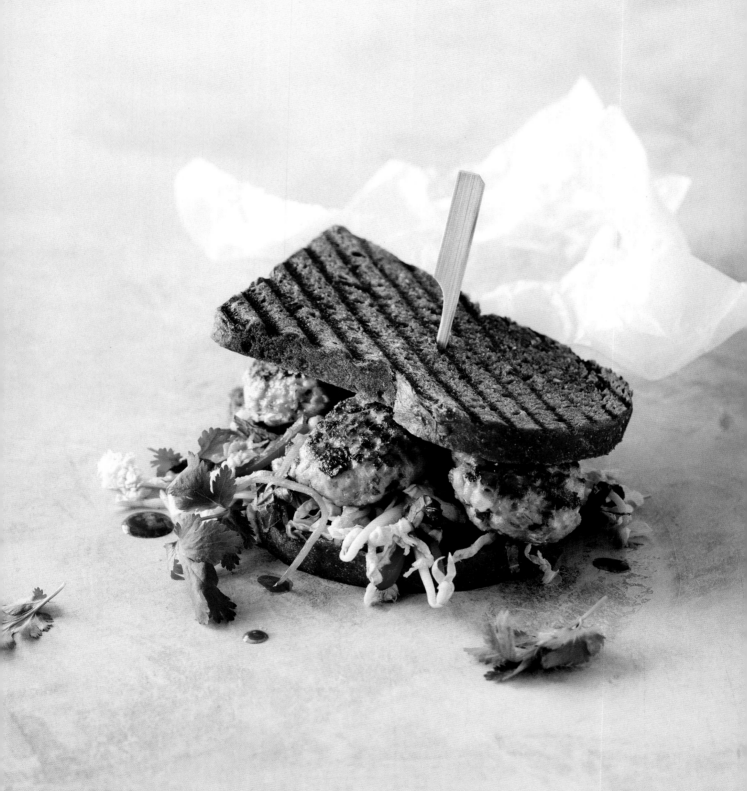

Vietnamese chicken meatball *and* Asian slaw sandwiches

SERVES 4
PREPARATION 25 minutes
COOKING 25 minutes

8 slices gluten-free wholegrain bread
coriander leaves, to serve

VIETNAMESE CHICKEN MEATBALLS
olive oil spray, for cooking
2 sticks celery, finely chopped
400 g minced chicken
1 spring onion (green top only),
    finely chopped
small handful coriander leaves,
    finely chopped
2 teaspoons tamari (gluten-free
    soy sauce)
1 egg white

ASIAN SLAW
1 cup (80 g) shredded Chinese
    cabbage (wombok)
½ cup (40 g) bean sprouts
1 carrot, coarsely grated
½ red capsicum, seeded
    and thinly sliced
small handful mint leaves, thinly sliced
2 teaspoons sesame oil
2 teaspoons tamari (gluten-free
    soy sauce)
½ teaspoon pure maple syrup
    (optional)

To make the meatballs, heat a non-stick heavy-based frying pan over low–medium heat, then spray with olive oil. Cook the celery with 1 tablespoon water for 3 minutes or until softened. Transfer to a large bowl and set aside to cool. Add the remaining ingredients and stir until well combined. Form the mixture into 16 meatballs (or 8 patties).

Heat the frying pan over medium heat and spray with olive oil. Working in batches, cook the meatballs (or patties), turning occasionally, for 8–10 minutes or until cooked through and golden, spraying with more olive oil if necessary to prevent sticking. (Patties may take a little longer, so reduce the heat to low–medium, if necessary, and continue to cook for another 1–2 minutes per side or until cooked through.)

Meanwhile, to make the slaw, place the cabbage, bean sprouts, carrot, capsicum and mint in a bowl and stir to mix well. Place the sesame oil, tamari and maple syrup in a small bowl and stir to combine. Add to the slaw and toss to coat.

Toast the bread. Top four of the slices with one-quarter of the slaw, then add 4 of the meatballs (or 2 of the patties), scatter with coriander leaves and pop the other toast slice on top. Serve immediately.

4 G FIBRE PER SERVE — LOW FODMAP

UNITS PER SERVE ❋ BREADS AND CEREALS **2** ❋ PROTEIN **1** ❋ FRUIT **0** ❋ VEGETABLES **1** ❋ DAIRY **0** ❋ FATS AND OILS **0.5**

Poached chicken waldorf sandwiches

SERVES 4
PREPARATION 15 minutes, plus standing time
COOKING 20 minutes

⅓ cup (80 g) lactose-free natural
    yoghurt, plus extra if needed
1 teaspoon Dijon mustard
1 small stick celery, finely chopped
2 tablespoons walnuts, finely chopped
1 tablespoon finely chopped
    flat-leaf parsley leaves
8 small seedless green grapes,
    thinly sliced
lemon juice, for squeezing
8 slices sourdough spelt bread
4 butter or inner iceberg lettuce
    leaves, shredded
handful rocket leaves

POACHED CHICKEN
4 gluten-free, FODMAP-friendly
    vegetable stock cubes, dissolved
    in 2 cups (500 ml) boiling water,
    plus extra if needed
4 black peppercorns
1 spring onion (green top only),
    thinly sliced
2 sprigs flat-leaf parsley
400 g chicken breast fillets

To poach the chicken, place the stock, peppercorns, spring onion and parsley in a small heavy-based saucepan and bring to the boil over high heat, then reduce the heat to medium and simmer for 5 minutes. Add the chicken breast, reduce the heat to low and cook for 15 minutes or until the chicken is cooked through. Remove from the heat, cover and leave to stand for 10 minutes. Transfer to a plate and, when cool enough to handle, thinly slice or cut into 5 mm dice.

Place the yoghurt, mustard, celery, walnuts, parsley and grapes in a bowl and add a squeeze of lemon juice to taste. Add the chicken, season with freshly ground black pepper and mix to coat well; add an extra 1–2 teaspoons yoghurt if a smoother mixture is preferred.

Place 4 slices of the bread on a chopping board and top each one with one-quarter of the lettuce and rocket, then add one-quarter of the chicken mixture. Top with the remaining bread slices, cut in half or into thirds and serve.

4 G FIBRE PER SERVE | **LOW FODMAP**

UNITS PER SERVE ❋ BREADS AND CEREALS **2** ❋ PROTEIN **1** ❋ FRUIT **0** ❋ VEGETABLES **0.5** ❋ DAIRY **0.5** ❋ FATS AND OILS **1.5**

Tuna *and* roasted vegetable salad *with* creamy Dijon dressing

SERVES 4
PREPARATION 20 minutes
COOKING 20 minutes, plus cooling time

1 cup (135 g) chopped unpeeled
   sweet potato
2 baby (finger) eggplants, sliced
1 zucchini, sliced
1 tablespoon garlic-infused olive oil
1 tablespoon rosemary leaves or
   ½ teaspoon dried rosemary
1 x 400 g tin tuna chunks in springwater,
   drained, thickly flaked
1 cup baby rocket leaves
1 tablespoon pumpkin seeds
   (pepitas), toasted
8 slices gluten-free chia and sunflower
   bread, toasted

CREAMY DIJON DRESSING

½ cup (120 g) lactose-free
   natural yoghurt
2 teaspoons Dijon mustard
2 tablespoons white wine vinegar
2 tablespoons finely chopped
   flat-leaf parsley leaves

Preheat the oven to 220°C (200°C fan-forced) and line a large baking tray with baking paper.

Place the sweet potato, eggplant and zucchini on the prepared tray. Drizzle with olive oil, sprinkle with rosemary and season to taste with freshly ground black pepper. Toss together to coat well, then roast for 20 minutes or until the vegetables are cooked and caramelised. Cool on the tray for 10 minutes, then transfer to a large heatproof bowl.

Meanwhile, to make the dressing, whisk together all the ingredients in a bowl and season to taste with freshly ground black pepper.

Add the tuna, rocket and pumpkin seeds to the vegetables and toss gently to combine. Divide evenly among 4 serving plates, spoon over the dressing and serve with toasted bread alongside.

Sweet potato is low-FODMAP in small quantities (up to ½ cup); more than this is high-FODMAP.

3 G FIBRE PER SERVE   **LOW FODMAP**   **GOOD SOURCE OF RESISTANT STARCH**

UNITS PER SERVE ❈ BREADS AND CEREALS **2** ❈ PROTEIN **1** ❈ FRUIT **0** ❈ VEGETABLES **1** ❈ DAIRY **0.5** ❈ FATS AND OILS **1.25**

Green tapenade *and* vegetable melt

SERVES 4
PREPARATION 20 minutes
COOKING 15 minutes

400 g chicken tenderloins,
    halved through centre
½ small eggplant, cut into 4 rounds
1 zucchini, halved crossways, then cut
    lengthways into 3 mm thick slices
8 slices gluten-free chia
    and sunflower bread or
    gluten-free seeded bread
1 large tomato, sliced into thin rounds
100 g mozzarella, grated

GREEN TAPENADE
1 cup baby spinach leaves
80 g pitted Sicilian green olives
1 tablespoon pumpkin seeds
    (pepitas), toasted
finely grated zest and juice of
    1 small lemon
2 teaspoons garlic-infused olive oil

To make the green tapenade, place all the ingredients in a small food processor and blend until smooth, adding a little water if required to loosen it. Season to taste with freshly ground black pepper.

Heat a large chargrill pan over high heat. Add the chicken and cook for 4 minutes on each side or until cooked and golden, then transfer to a plate. Add the eggplant and zucchini slices and cook for 2 minutes on each side or until just tender.

Preheat the oven grill to high. Grill the bread on one side for 30 seconds or until golden. Turn half the slices over and leave them on the grill tray. Remove the remaining slices and spread the uncooked side with some of the green tapenade, then top with the warm chargrilled chicken, vegetables, tomato slices and mozzarella. Return them to the grill and cook for 30 seconds. Remove the plain bread slices and continue to grill the topped bread for 1–2 minutes or until the cheese has melted.

Dollop the remaining tapenade over the melts and place the toasted bread slices on top. Serve warm.

9 G FIBRE PER SERVE   LOW FODMAP   GOOD SOURCE OF RESISTANT STARCH

UNITS PER SERVE   ❋ BREADS AND CEREALS **2**   ❋ PROTEIN **1**   ❋ FRUIT **0**   ❋ VEGETABLES **1**   ❋ DAIRY **1**   ❋ FATS AND OILS **0.5**

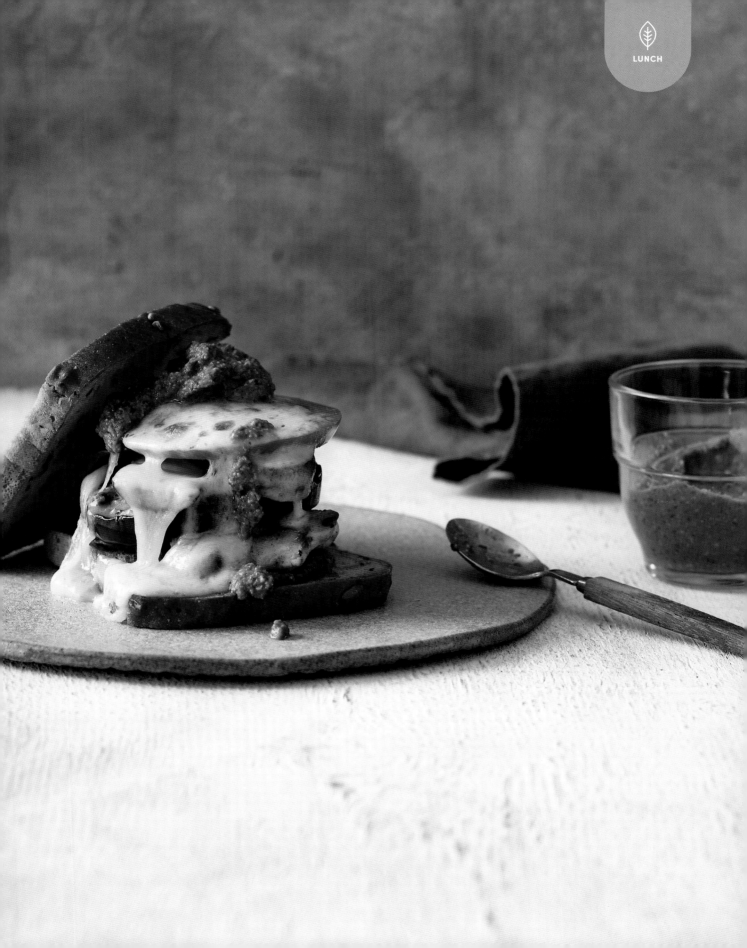

Lunchbowls 4 ways

South-western prawn *and* green bean rice bowl

SERVES 4
PREPARATION 20 minutes
COOKING 15 minutes, plus rice cooking time

120 g green beans, trimmed

2 cups (370 g) cooked basmati rice (see page 41)

small handful roughly chopped coriander leaves, plus extra sprigs to serve (optional)

400 g cooked, peeled king prawns, with tails intact

200 g cherry or grape tomatoes, halved

1 baby cos lettuce, trimmed and quartered lengthways

120 g salt-reduced low-fat feta, crumbled

30 g toasted pecans, roughly chopped

lime wedges, to serve

Cook the green beans in a saucepan of simmering water for 3 minutes or until cooked, then drain and transfer to a bowl. Add the rice and coriander and stir gently to mix through.

Divide the rice and bean mixture among 4 bowls, then top each bowl with one-quarter of the prawns, tomato, lettuce and feta. Scatter with pecans, extra coriander sprigs, if desired, then serve with lime wedges to the side.

5 G FIBRE PER SERVE **LOW FODMAP** **GOOD SOURCE OF RESISTANT STARCH**

UNITS PER SERVE ✳ BREADS AND CEREALS **2** ✳ PROTEIN **1** ✳ FRUIT **0** ✳ VEGETABLES **4** ✳ DAIRY **0.5** ✳ FATS AND OILS **1**

Sukiyaki beef bowl

SERVES 4
PREPARATION 20 minutes, plus marinating time
COOKING 10 minutes, plus rice cooking time

1 × 400 g beef eye fillet, all visible
    fat removed, thinly sliced

3 teaspoons tamari (gluten-free
    soy sauce)

1 teaspoon pure maple syrup

1 teaspoon finely grated ginger

2 teaspoons garlic-infused olive oil

2 sticks celery, halved lengthways
    and thinly sliced on the diagonal

1 small red capsicum, seeded and
    thinly sliced

100 g Chinese cabbage (wombok),
    shredded

3 zucchini, cut into thick matchsticks

2 cups (370 g) cooked basmati rice
    (see page 41)

Place the beef, tamari, maple syrup and ginger in a bowl, stir to coat. Cover with plastic film and marinate in the refrigerator for at least 30 minutes.

Heat a wok over high heat and add one-third of the oil. When the surface of the oil shimmers slightly, dd half of the beef and cook on one side for 1 minute or until lightly browned, then turn the beef and cook on the other side for another minute or until browned. Transfer to a bowl. Add another one-third of the oil and repeat with the remaining beef.

Place the remaining oil in the wok, then add the celery, capsicum, cabbage and zucchini and stir-fry for 2–3 minutes or until the vegetables are tender. Add to the bowl with the beef.

Divide the rice among 4 bowls and then top each one with one-quarter each of the beef and vegetable mixture (including any juices). Serve immediately.

To take these from the lunchbox to the dinner table, simply double the amount of protein, halve the rice and add 1 cup (120 g) cooked and drained frozen peas to boost the resistant starch. Serve with 2 cups leafy green salad alongside.

4 G FIBRE PER SERVE   **LOW FODMAP**

UNITS PER SERVE ❋ BREADS AND CEREALS **1** ❋ PROTEIN **1** ❋ FRUIT **0** ❋ VEGETABLES **2.5** ❋ DAIRY **0** ❋ FATS AND OILS **0**

Broad bean *and* pea falafel bowl *with* whipped feta

SERVES 4
PREPARATION 30 minutes, plus refrigerating time
COOKING 25 minutes

2 Lebanese cucumbers, shaved with
    a vegetable peeler
250 g grape or cherry tomatoes, halved
2 baby cos lettuces, leaves separated
    and torn
4 slices rye pumpernickel, toasted and
    torn into bite-sized pieces

BROAD BEAN AND PEA FALAFELS

375 g frozen broad beans
¼ cup (30 g) frozen peas
1 × 400 g tin salt-reduced chickpeas,
    drained and rinsed
¼ small onion, roughly chopped
small handful roughly chopped
    coriander leaves
small handful roughly chopped
    flat-leaf parsley leaves
1 clove garlic, crushed
2 teaspoons finely grated lemon zest
1 teaspoon ground cumin
1 teaspoon sweet paprika
1½ tablespoons plain flour
olive oil spray, for cooking

WHIPPED FETA

100 g salt-reduced low-fat feta
2½ tablespoons (50 g) reduced-fat
    natural Greek-style yoghurt
sumac, for sprinkling (optional)

To make the falafels, cook the broad beans in a saucepan of simmering water for 3 minutes or until cooked. Drain, run under cold water, then double-peel when cool enough to handle and transfer to a food processor or blender. Cook the peas in a saucepan of simmering water until tender, then drain and add to the food processor or blender. Add the chickpeas, onion, coriander, parsley, garlic, lemon zest, cumin and paprika and process to form a coarse paste; take care not to over-process. Stir in the flour then, using wet hands, divide the mixture into 24 even portions. Roll each one into a ball, place on a baking tray lined with baking paper and gently flatten; they should be about 2 cm wide and 1 cm thick. Cover with plastic film and refrigerate for 30 minutes to firm up.

To make the whipped feta, place the feta and yoghurt in a small food processor and process until smooth and well combined. Transfer to a small bowl and sprinkle with sumac, if using.

Heat a large non-stick heavy-based frying pan over medium heat and spray with olive oil. Working in batches, pan-fry the falafels over low heat for 4–5 minutes on each side or until golden brown.

Divide the cucumber, tomato, lettuce and bread among 4 bowls and top with 3 falafels each. Finish with a spoonful of whipped feta, then serve the remaining whipped feta alongside.

This will make twice as many falafels as you'll need for this dish, so you can either store the leftover falafels and enjoy them the next day, or halve the quantities to make a smaller batch.

17 G FIBRE PER SERVE **GOOD SOURCE OF RESISTANT STARCH**

UNITS PER SERVE ❋ BREADS AND CEREALS **2** ❋ PROTEIN **1** ❋ FRUIT **0** ❋ VEGETABLES **1** ❋ DAIRY **1** ❋ FATS AND OILS **0**

Sesame haloumi, chargrilled vegetable *and* sumac chickpea bowl

SERVES 4
PREPARATION 20 minutes
COOKING 25 minutes, plus sweet potato cooking time

¾ cup (135 g) McKenzie's SuperBlend Fibre 'Freekeh, Lentils & Beans' (available in the legume section of larger supermarkets)

olive oil spray, for cooking

1 sweet potato (600 g), cut widthways into 5 mm thick slices, steamed and chilled overnight (see page 41)

1 large red capsicum, seeded and cut into thick slices

2 zucchini, thinly sliced lengthways

2 Lebanese eggplants, halved lengthways

1 red onion, cut into wedges

250 g grape or cherry tomatoes

sesame seeds, for coating

100 g haloumi, cut widthways into 4 slices

150 g rocket leaves

SUMAC CHICKPEAS

olive oil spray, for cooking

1 × 400 g tin salt-reduced chickpeas, drained, rinsed and patted dry

½ teaspoon sumac

Fill a heavy-based saucepan with water and bring to the boil over high heat. Add the freekeh, lentil and bean mixture, then reduce the heat to medium and cook, stirring occasionally, for 15 minutes or until tender. Drain, transfer to a bowl and set aside.

Meanwhile, heat a chargrill pan or large heavy-based saucepan over medium–high heat and spray with olive oil. Working in batches, chargrill the sweet potato for 2–3 minutes or until heated through and the capsicum for 4–5 minutes or until tender and chargrill marks appear. Transfer each to a plate and set aside. Repeat with the zucchini, eggplant and onion, then chargrill the tomatoes for 2 minutes on each side or until just blistered.

To make the sumac chickpeas, heat a small heavy-based saucepan over medium heat, then spray with olive oil. Add the chickpeas and sumac and stir to combine, then cook for 2–3 minutes or until heated through.

Just before serving, spread a layer of sesame seeds on a plate, coat the haloumi slices on both sides and spray with olive oil. Chargrill or pan-fry the haloumi for 1–2 minutes on each side until just golden.

Divide the freekeh mixture among 4 bowls, then top each with one-quarter of the chargrilled vegetables, sumac chickpeas, rocket and haloumi and serve.

24 G FIBRE PER SERVE · GOOD SOURCE OF RESISTANT STARCH

UNITS PER SERVE ❋ BREADS AND CEREALS **2** ❋ PROTEIN **1** ❋ FRUIT **0** ❋ VEGETABLES **2** ❋ DAIRY **1** ❋ FATS AND OILS **0**

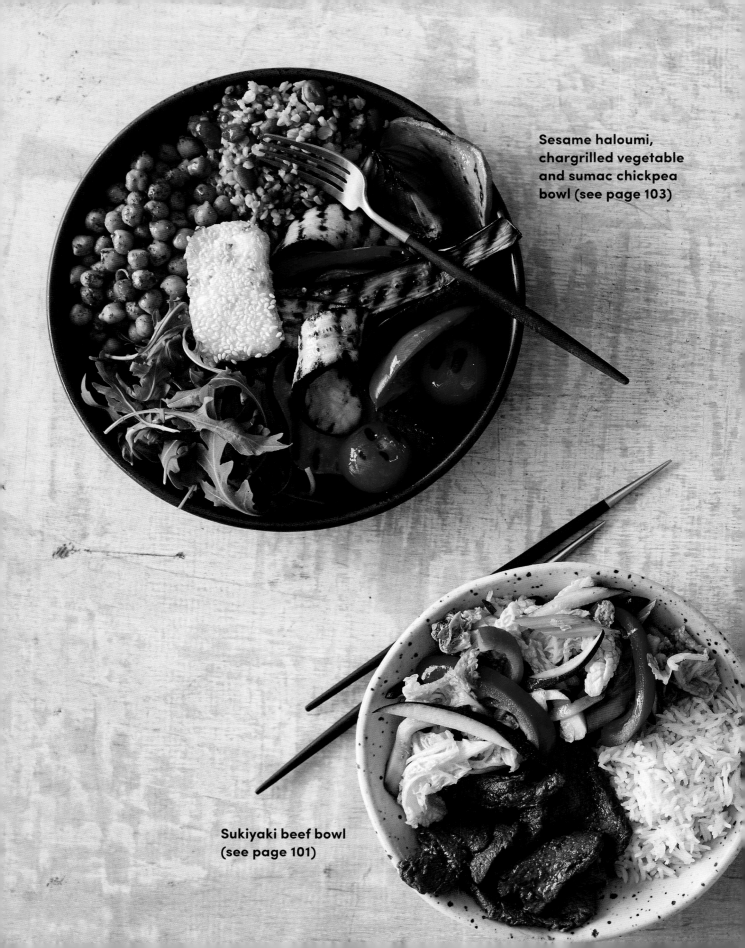

Sesame haloumi, chargrilled vegetable and sumac chickpea bowl (see page 103)

Sukiyaki beef bowl (see page 101)

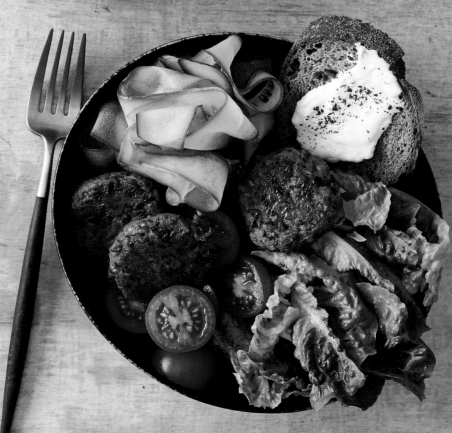

South-western prawn
and green bean rice bowl
(see page 100)

Broad bean and pea falafel bowl
with whipped feta (see page 102)

Chicken Lunchbowls 4 ways

Chicken enchilada bowl

SERVES 4
PREPARATION 15 minutes, plus standing time
COOKING 30 minutes, plus rice cooking time

2 red capsicums, seeded and quartered
2 teaspoons garlic-infused olive oil
2 sticks celery, finely chopped
1 teaspoon chilli powder
1 teaspoon ground cumin
¼ teaspoon smoked sweet paprika,
　or to taste
1 × 400 g tin salt-reduced
　chopped tomatoes
400 g chicken breast fillets
2 cups (370 g) cooked basmati rice
　(see page 41)
100 g reduced-fat cheddar, grated
80 g brazil nuts, toasted and
　roughly chopped
150 g mixed salad leaves

Preheat the oven grill to high and line a baking tray with baking paper. Grill the capsicum, skin-side up, for 15 minutes or until tender and charred. Transfer to a bowl, cover with plastic film and leave to steam for 10 minutes, then peel off the skin and cut into wide strips.

Meanwhile, heat a deep heavy-based frying pan with a lid over medium heat and add the oil. Add the celery and cook for 3 minutes or until softened but not coloured, then add the chilli powder, cumin and paprika and stir to mix. Stir in the tomatoes and ¾ cup (180 ml) water and bring to a simmer over medium–high heat. Add the chicken, then cover and cook over medium heat for 25 minutes or until the chicken is cooked through. Using 2 forks, shred the chicken, then turn to coat in the sauce. Season to taste with freshly ground black pepper.

Divide the rice among 4 bowls, then top each bowl with one-quarter of the chicken enchilada mixture. Finish with one-quarter of the capsicum strips, cheese, brazil nuts and salad leaves and serve immediately.

8 G FIBRE PER SERVE　　LOW FODMAP

UNITS PER SERVE BREADS AND CEREALS **2** ✱ PROTEIN **1** ✱ FRUIT **0** ✱ VEGETABLES **1** ✱ DAIRY **0** ✱ FATS AND OILS **3**

Thai coriander, turmeric *and* pepper chicken bowl

SERVES 4
PREPARATION 20 minutes, plus marinating time
COOKING 30 minutes, plus rice cooking time

3 coriander roots and stems, well
    washed and finely chopped
1 clove garlic, finely chopped
1 teaspoon ground turmeric
¼ teaspoon freshly ground
    black pepper, or to taste
3 teaspoons extra virgin olive oil
400 g chicken breast fillets,
    halved widthways and cut
    into bite-sized pieces
2 bunches baby bok choy,
    halved or quartered
125 g baby corn, larger ones
    halved lengthways
24 snow peas, halved on the diagonal
150 g snake beans, cut into 2 cm lengths
olive oil spray, for cooking
2 tablespoons raw cashews
1 teaspoon fish sauce
2 cups (370 g) cooked basmati
    rice (see page 41)

Combine the coriander, garlic, turmeric, pepper and olive oil in a small bowl. Place the chicken in a shallow bowl and spread the coriander marinade over to coat evenly. Cover with plastic film and marinate in the refrigerator for at least 15 minutes.

Meanwhile, working in batches, steam the vegetables in a steamer basket over a saucepan of simmering water: steam the bok choy for 2 minutes or until wilted, and the baby corn, snow peas and snake beans for 3 minutes or until tender but crisp. Set aside.

Heat a non-stick heavy-based frying pan over medium heat. Working in batches, add the chicken to the pan, then cook for 3–4 minutes until a crust forms and the outside is golden. Carefully turn and cook on the other side for another 2–3 minutes or until a crust forms and the chicken is cooked through; reduce the heat to low–medium if necessary so the chicken cooks through and the outside is slightly charred. Transfer to a plate, then add the cashews to the pan and cook, stirring, for 2 minutes or until lightly toasted. Add to the plate of chicken.

Add the vegetables and fish sauce to the pan and stir for 30 seconds to coat in the fish sauce. Divide the rice among 4 bowls and top each one with one-quarter of the chicken and cashew mixture and one-quarter of the vegetables. Serve immediately.

10 G FIBRE PER SERVE   **GOOD SOURCE OF RESISTANT STARCH**

UNITS PER SERVE ✻ BREADS AND CEREALS **2** ✻ PROTEIN **1** ✻ FRUIT **0** ✻ VEGETABLES **1** ✻ DAIRY **0** ✻ FATS AND OILS **2**

Teriyaki chicken rice bowl

SERVES 4
PREPARATION 20 minutes, plus marinating time
COOKING 25 minutes, plus rice cooking time

400 g chicken breast fillets, halved
    widthways and cut into 1.5 cm cubes
2 teaspoons pure maple syrup
1 tablespoon sake or dry sherry
2 teaspoons tamari (gluten-free
    soy sauce)
1 teaspoon finely grated ginger
sesame oil, for drizzling
olive oil spray, for cooking
1 tablespoon sesame seeds,
    lightly toasted
1 bunch (3 pieces) baby bok choy,
    leaves separated
1 red capsicum, seeded and thinly sliced
2 spring onions (green tops only),
    cut into 1.5 cm lengths
2 cups (370 g) cooked basmati rice
    (see page 41)

Place the chicken in a glass bowl. Combine the maple syrup, sake or sherry, tamari and ginger in a small bowl and stir to combine, then add a few drops of sesame oil. Add to the chicken and stir to coat well, then cover with plastic film and refrigerate until required.

Heat a wok over high heat, then spray with olive oil. Working in batches, cook the chicken for 2–3 minutes; do not stir-fry. Carefully turn each piece and cook for another 2–3 minutes until cooked through. Transfer to a bowl and cover loosely with foil to keep warm, while you cook the remaining chicken and the vegetables. Add any remaining marinade to the wok when cooking the last batch of chicken, then bring to the boil to cook it through. Scatter the sesame seeds over the chicken.

Stir-fry the bok choy and 2 tablespoons water first for 30 seconds, then add the capsicum and spring onion and stir-fry for 1–2 minutes or until tender but still crisp, transfer to a separate bowl.

Divide the rice among 4 bowls, then top each one with one-quarter of the chicken and vegetables. Serve immediately.

5 G FIBRE PER SERVE   LOW FODMAP

UNITS PER SERVE ✳ BREADS AND CEREALS **2** ✳ PROTEIN **1** ✳ FRUIT **0** ✳ VEGETABLES **1** ✳ DAIRY **0** ✳ FATS AND OILS **1.25**

Bang bang chicken rice bowl

SERVES 4
PREPARATION 20 minutes
COOKING 20 minutes, plus rice cooking time

3 gluten-free, FODMAP-friendly
    chicken stock cubes, dissolved in
    2 cups (500 ml) boiling water
1 star anise
1 teaspoon Sichuan peppercorns
1 cm piece ginger, crushed
400 g chicken breast fillets
150 g green beans, trimmed
2 Lebanese cucumbers, cut into
    thin batons
1 carrot, cut into thin batons
1 pale inner stalk celery, cut into
    thin batons
½ iceberg lettuce or ¼ Chinese cabbage
    (wombok), shredded
2 spring onions (green tops only),
    finely chopped
2 cups (370 g) cooked basmati rice
    (see page 41)

CASHEW–TAHINI DRESSING
1 teaspoon garlic-infused olive oil
2 tablespoons unsalted cashew butter
1 teaspoon tahini
1–2 teaspoons lime juice, or to taste
1½–2 tablespoons boiling water
2 teaspoons tamari (gluten-free
    soy sauce)

Place the stock, star anise, Sichuan peppercorns and ginger in a small heavy-based saucepan and bring to the boil over high heat. Add the chicken and a little water if necessary to ensure it is covered, then return to a simmer. Reduce the heat to low–medium and simmer for 12 minutes or until the chicken is cooked through. Remove from the heat, cover and leave to rest in the poaching liquid while you prepare the salad.

Cook the green beans in a saucepan of simmering water for 3 minutes or until tender but still crisp, then drain and set aside.

To make the dressing, place all the ingredients together in a small bowl and stir until smooth and well combined. Set aside until required.

Cut the chicken into thick slices or shred into bite-sized pieces, using 2 forks; discard the cooking liquid.

Place the green beans, cucumber, carrot, celery and lettuce or cabbage in a bowl and gently toss to combine. Add a spoonful of the dressing and toss gently to mix through. (Alternatively, place each one in a separate pile on top of the rice in each bowl.)

Divide the rice among 4 bowls, then top each one with one-quarter of the chicken and one-quarter of the salad. Drizzle the remaining dressing evenly over the chicken, then scatter with spring onion and serve immediately.

Instead of poaching chicken breast fillets, you could use 400 g peeled, cooked king prawns for an even faster lunch option.

6 G FIBRE PER SERVE **GOOD SOURCE OF RESISTANT STARCH**

UNITS PER SERVE ❋ BREADS AND CEREALS **2** ❋ PROTEIN **1** ❋ FRUIT **0** ❋ VEGETABLES **2** ❋ DAIRY **0** ❋ FATS AND OILS **2**

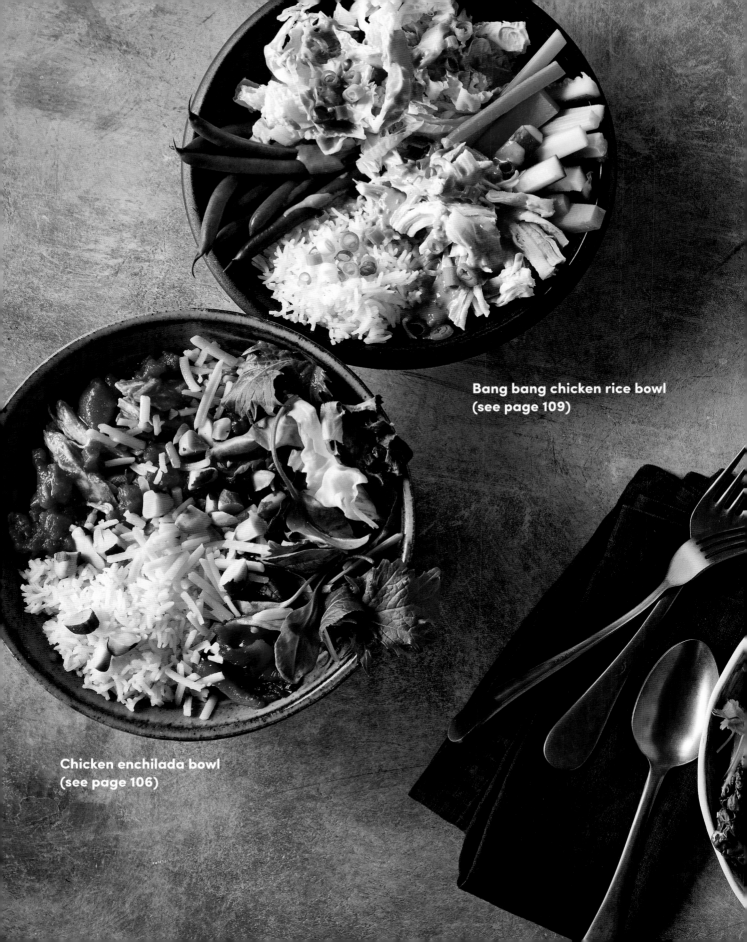

Bang bang chicken rice bowl
(see page 109)

Chicken enchilada bowl
(see page 106)

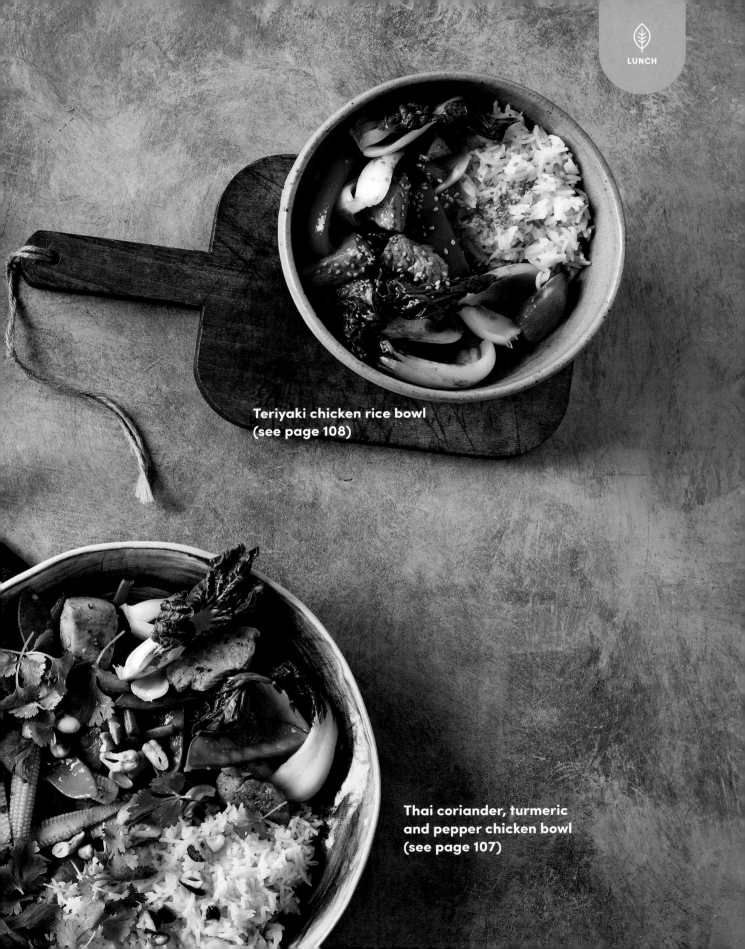

Teriyaki chicken rice bowl
(see page 108)

Thai coriander, turmeric
and pepper chicken bowl
(see page 107)

Sushi Lunchbowls 4 ways

Sushi rice

1⅓ cups (265 g) sushi rice
¼ cup (60 ml) rice vinegar
2 teaspoons sugar
4 sheets nori, thinly sliced or shredded

Steam the rice according to the packet instructions, then immediately spread out on a baking tray. Combine the vinegar and sugar and pour evenly over the rice, then set aside to cool.

As soon as the rice is cool, scatter with the nori and it's ready to use in the following recipes.

In place of the sushi rice, you could also use ½ cup (100 g) long-grain brown rice and ½ cup (100 g) pearl barley and cook together in 1½ cups water for 30-35 minutes.

Sashimi sushi bowl

SERVES 4
PREPARATION 10 minutes
COOKING 3 minutes, plus rice cooking time

1 quantity Sushi Rice (see opposite page)
1 × 400 g piece sashimi-grade salmon or tuna
    (or half each), thinly sliced
4 radishes, shaved
100 g mizuna or wild rocket leaves
100 g green beans, blanched and drained
seaweed salad (available from sushi stores,
    fishmongers and the sushi section of larger
    supermarkets), to serve (optional)
furikake, for sprinkling (optional)

Divide all the ingredients among 4 small shallow
bowls and serve immediately.

6 G FIBRE PER SERVE

UNITS PER SERVE ❀ BREADS AND CEREALS **2** ❀ PROTEIN **1** ❀ FRUIT **0** ❀ VEGETABLES **1** ❀ DAIRY **0** ❀ FATS AND OILS **1**

California roll bowl

SERVES 4
PREPARATION 15 minutes
COOKING Nil, plus rice cooking time

1 quantity Sushi Rice (see opposite page)
400 g cooked crabmeat (available from fishmongers)
2 Lebanese cucumbers, halved lengthways, seeded
    and cut into julienne or 1 cm dice
1 small carrot, cut into julienne or coarsely grated
80 g avocado, thinly sliced or cut into 1 cm dice
1 spring onion, finely chopped
sesame seeds, for sprinkling

Divide all the ingredients among 4 small shallow
bowls and serve immediately.

5 G FIBRE PER SERVE

UNITS PER SERVE ❀ BREADS AND CEREALS **2** ❀ PROTEIN **1** ❀ FRUIT **0** ❀ VEGETABLES **2** ❀ DAIRY **0** ❀ FATS AND OILS **0**

Vegetarian sushi bowl

SERVES 4
PREPARATION 10 minutes
COOKING 15–20 minutes, plus rice cooking time

1 quantity Sushi Rice (see page 112)
8 eggs, soft-boiled (see opposite) or
    4 eggs, cooked as an omelette
    (see page 188)
1 quantity pan-fried tofu (see page 188)
1 cup (120 g) frozen peas, boiled
    and drained
100 g podded frozen broad beans,
    boiled and drained
100 g red cabbage, shredded
100 g button mushrooms, thinly sliced
12 snow peas, shredded

Divide all the ingredients among 4 small shallow bowls and serve immediately.

11 G FIBRE PER SERVE

UNITS PER SERVE ✳ BREADS AND CEREALS **2** ✳ PROTEIN **1** ✳ FRUIT **0** ✳ VEGETABLES **1** ✳ DAIRY **0** ✳ FATS AND OILS **1**

Sesame egg *and* ginger zucchini quinoa sushi bowl

SERVES 4
PREPARATION 10 minutes
COOKING 10 minutes, plus quinoa cooking time

8 eggs
2 tablespoons sesame seeds
1 teaspoon cumin seeds
2 cups (370 g) cooked quinoa,
    cooled (made from 1 cup/190 g
    uncooked quinoa)
2 cups (150 g) baby spinach leaves
1 stick celery, cut into thin matchsticks

GINGER ZUCCHINI
1 zucchini, very thinly sliced into rounds
3 cm piece ginger, finely grated
¼ cup (60 ml) apple cider vinegar
2 teaspoons garlic-infused olive oil

To make the ginger zucchini, combine all the ingredients in a bowl. Set aside to quick-pickle, stirring occasionally.

Cook the eggs in a saucepan of boiling water for 4 minutes for soft-boiled or 6 minutes for hard-boiled. Remove and cool under cold running water, then peel away the shells and cut the eggs in half lengthways.

Meanwhile, combine the sesame seeds and cumin seeds in a small non-stick frying pan and toast over low heat for 1–2 minutes until golden and fragrant. Immediately transfer them to a bowl and leave to cool.

Sprinkle half the cut sides of the cooked eggs with the seed mixture to coat.

Toss together the quinoa, baby spinach and celery, then divide evenly among 4 serving bowls. Top with the seed-crusted eggs and spoon over the ginger zucchini.

5 G FIBRE PER SERVE   LOW FODMAP

UNITS PER SERVE ✳ BREADS AND CEREALS **2** ✳ PROTEIN **1** ✳ FRUIT **0** ✳ VEGETABLES **2** ✳ DAIRY **0** ✳ FATS AND OILS **0**

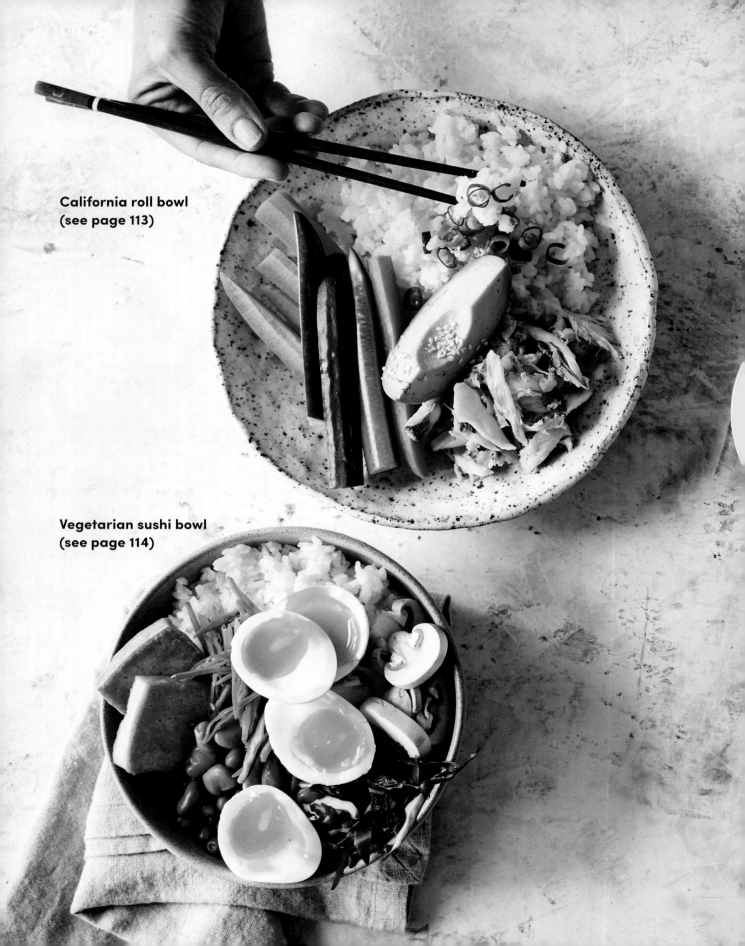

California roll bowl
(see page 113)

Vegetarian sushi bowl
(see page 114)

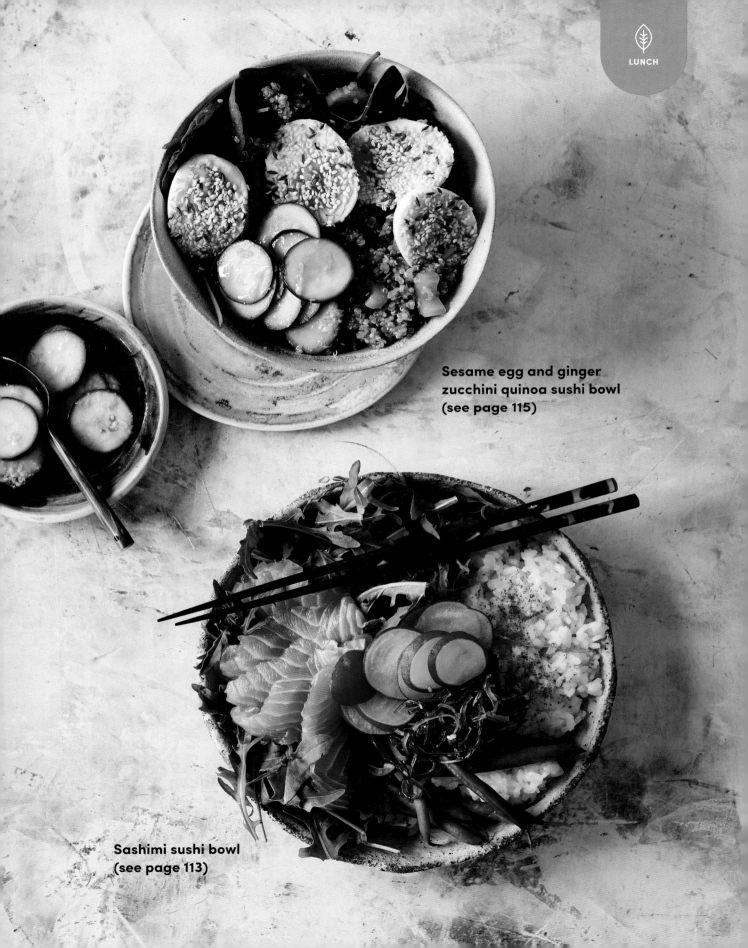

**Sesame egg and ginger
zucchini quinoa sushi bowl
(see page 115)**

**Sashimi sushi bowl
(see page 113)**

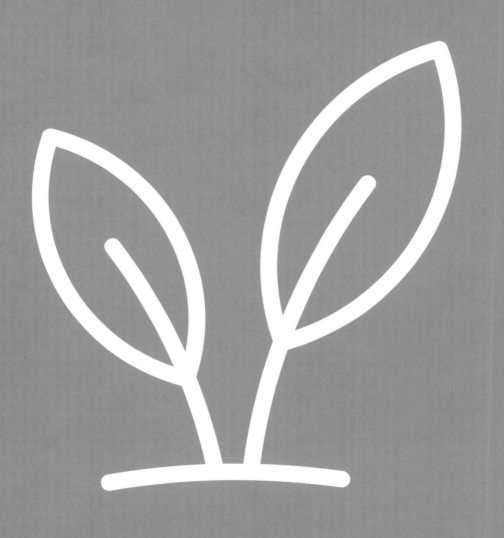

Seafood Mains

Cashew dukkah-crusted ocean trout *with* freekeh, lentil *and* watercress salad

SERVES 4
PREPARATION 30 minutes
COOKING 20 minutes

olive oil spray, for cooking
4 × 200 g ocean trout fillets, skin on
    and pin-boned
1 bunch asparagus, bases trimmed
1 bunch broccolini, bases trimmed
800 g reduced-fat natural Greek-style
    yoghurt mixed with 1 tablespoon
    ground cumin

FREEKEH, LENTIL AND WATERCRESS SALAD
1 stick cinnamon
1 wide strip orange zest
¾ cup (135 g) McKenzie's SuperBlend
    Fibre 'Freekeh, Lentils and Beans'
    (available in the legume section
    of larger supermarkets)
2 tablespoons orange juice
2 teaspoons extra virgin olive oil
1 teaspoon ground cumin
150 g green beans, trimmed
150 g sugar snap peas
1 bunch watercress, leaves picked
3 tablespoons chopped flat-leaf parsley
3 tablespoons roughly chopped mint

CASHEW DUKKAH
½ cup (80 g) raw cashews
¼ small red onion, finely chopped
3 tablespoons finely chopped
    flat-leaf parsley
3 tablespoons finely chopped mint
finely grated zest of 1 lemon

For the freekeh salad, place the cinnamon stick, orange zest and 540 ml water in a heavy-based saucepan and bring to the boil over high heat. Add the freekeh, lentil and bean mixture, then reduce the heat to medium and cook, stirring occasionally, for 15 minutes or until tender. Drain well, then remove and discard the cinnamon stick and orange zest. Transfer to a bowl and set aside. Combine the orange juice, olive oil and cumin in a small bowl and set aside. Steam the beans and sugar snap peas for 3 minutes or until tender but crisp. Set aside to cool.

Meanwhile, for the cashew dukkah, preheat the oven to 180°C (160°C fan-forced). Roast the cashews on a baking tray for 5–6 minutes until light golden, then pound using a mortar and pestle until coarsely crushed. Transfer to a shallow plate, then add the remaining ingredients and stir to combine. Set aside.

Heat a non-stick heavy-based frying pan over medium–high heat, then spray with olive oil. Add the ocean trout, skin-side down, and cook for 2–3 minutes until the skin is golden and crisp. Turn and cook for a further 2–3 minutes for medium or until cooked to your liking. Transfer, flesh-side down, to the plate with the cashew dukkah and press firmly to coat the surface. Set aside.

Steam the asparagus and broccolini for 3 minutes or until just tender. Set aside. Stir the reserved orange-juice dressing, beans, sugar snap peas, watercress and herbs through the freekeh mixture.

Divide the cumin yoghurt among 4 plates, then top with one-quarter of the freekeh salad. Add an ocean trout fillet and one-quarter of the asparagus and broccolini to each plate, then serve.

13 G FIBRE PER SERVE   GOOD SOURCE OF RESISTANT STARCH

UNITS PER SERVE ❋ BREADS AND CEREALS **1** ❋ PROTEIN **2** ❋ FRUIT **0** ❋ VEGETABLES **2** ❋ DAIRY **1** ❋ FATS AND OILS **2.5**

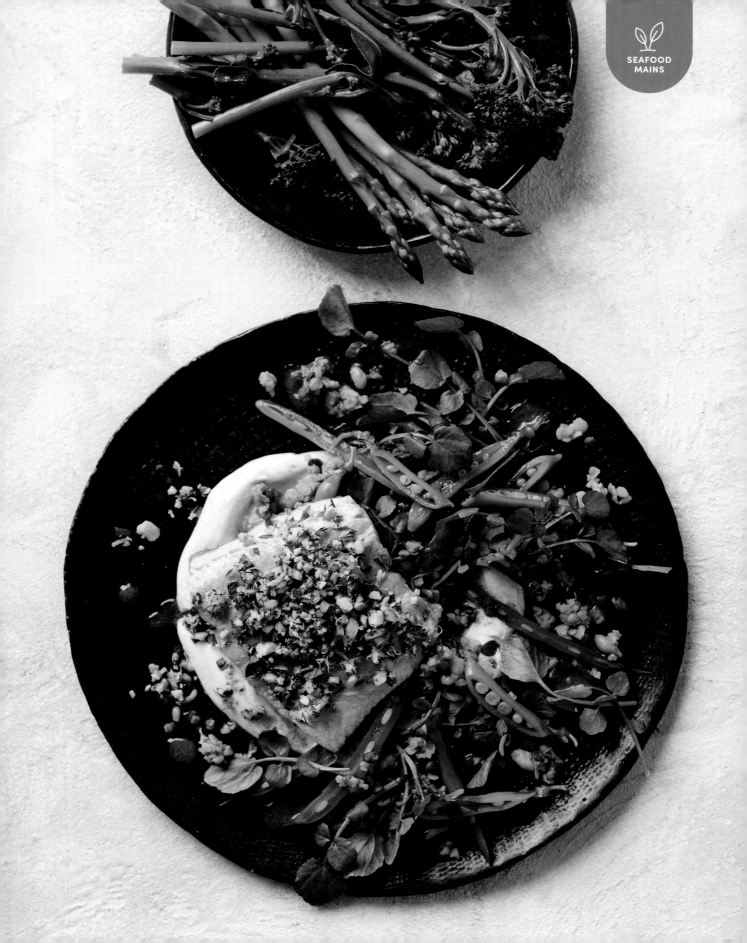

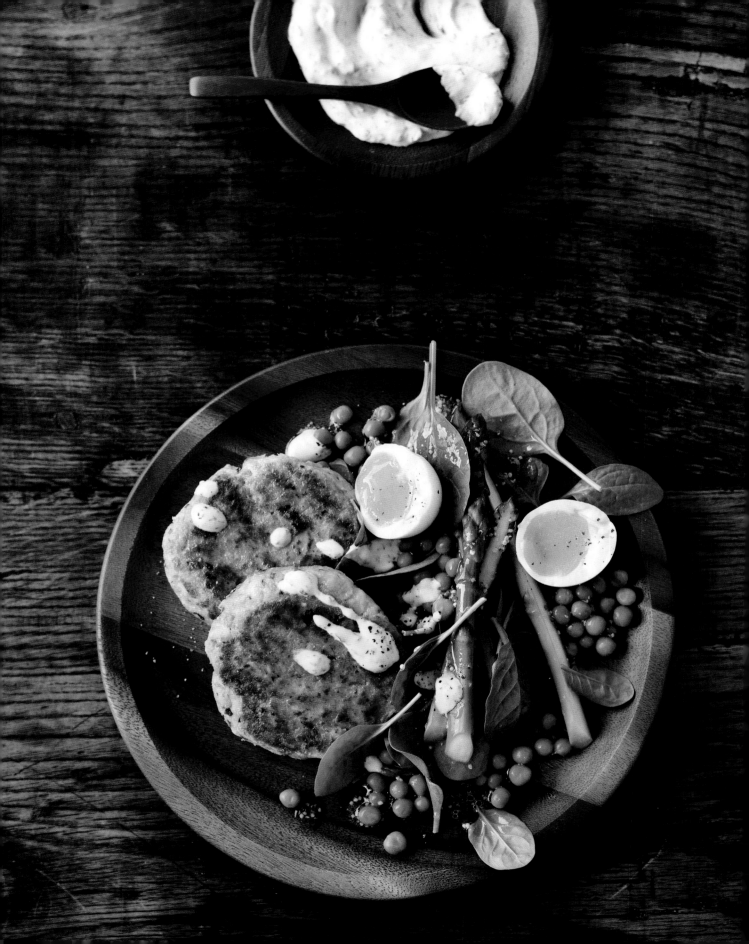

Salmon *and* cauliflower fishcakes *with* pea, spinach *and* asparagus salad

SERVES 4
PREPARATION 25 minutes, plus refrigerating time
COOKING 40 minutes, plus potato cooking time

1 small head cauliflower, trimmed and
cut into small florets
2 potatoes, quartered, steamed and
chilled overnight (see page 41)
545 g tinned salmon, drained, skin
and bones removed, flaked
¼ cup (35 g) plain flour,
plus extra for dusting
finely grated zest of 1 lemon
2 tablespoons finely chopped chives
2 tablespoons finely chopped
flat-leaf parsley leaves
olive oil spray, for cooking

PEA, SPINACH AND ASPARAGUS SALAD
4 eggs
1½ cups (180 g) frozen peas
1 bunch asparagus, bases trimmed
2 cups (150 g) baby spinach leaves,
stems trimmed
2 tablespoons lemon juice
1 teaspoon wholegrain mustard
1 tablespoon extra virgin olive oil

MINTED YOGHURT
100 g reduced-fat natural
Greek-style yoghurt
2 tablespoons finely chopped
mint leaves
1–2 teaspoons lemon juice, to taste

Steam the cauliflower for 6 minutes or until tender. Transfer to a food processor or blender and blend to form a chunky puree. Place in a bowl, add the potato and mash to combine. Stir in the salmon, flour, lemon zest, chives and parsley and mix to combine. Divide into 8 even portions, then shape into patties. Place on a baking tray lined with baking paper, cover with plastic film and refrigerate for 30 minutes to firm.

Meanwhile, to make the salad, boil the eggs in a saucepan of simmering water for 7 minutes for medium–soft. Drain, then peel and cut in half. Cook the peas in a saucepan of simmering water for 3 minutes or until tender, then drain and set aside. Blanch the asparagus in a saucepan of simmering water for 2 minutes or until tender but still crisp, then drain and set aside. Place the spinach leaves in a bowl, then add the cooled peas and asparagus. Mix the lemon juice, mustard and olive oil in a small bowl until well combined and emulsified, then set aside.

To make the minted yoghurt, mix the yoghurt and mint in a small bowl, then stir in the lemon juice to taste. Cover with plastic film and refrigerate until required.

Heat a non-stick heavy-based frying pan over medium heat and spray with olive oil. Dust the salmon cakes lightly in flour, shaking to remove the excess. Pan-fry, in batches if necessary, for 4–5 minutes on each side until golden brown and warmed through; reduce the heat to low–medium if necessary.

Add the dressing to the salad and toss gently to coat. Divide the salad among 4 plates and top with one egg and 2 salmon cakes each, then serve with the minted yoghurt alongside.

11 G FIBRE PER SERVE | **GOOD SOURCE OF RESISTANT STARCH**

UNITS PER SERVE ❋ BREADS AND CEREALS **1** ❋ PROTEIN **2** ❋ FRUIT **0** ❋ VEGETABLES **2** ❋ DAIRY **0.5** ❋ FATS AND OILS **1**

Crisp-skinned salmon *with* brown rice, green bean *and* zucchini salad

SERVES 4
PREPARATION 15 minutes
COOKING 10 minutes, plus rice cooking time

olive oil spray, for cooking
4 × 200 g salmon fillets,
    skin on and pin-boned
black or white sesame seeds,
    to serve (optional)
lemon wedges, to serve

BROWN RICE, GREEN BEAN AND
ZUCCHINI SALAD
300 g green beans, trimmed
4 zucchini, peeled into long thin
    ribbons using a vegetable peeler
1 cup (185 g) cooked brown rice
    (see page 41)
¼ cup (40 g) unsalted roasted cashews
1 tablespoon sunflower seeds

DRESSING
3 teaspoons lemon juice
3 teaspoons tamari (gluten-free
    soy sauce)
1 teaspoon pure maple syrup

Add the green beans to a large saucepan of boiling water and cook for 3 minutes or until just tender. Drain and place under cold running water to cool. Drain well and set aside in a large bowl. Carefully stir through the zucchini ribbons and the cooked rice.

To make the dressing, place all the ingredients in a small bowl and stir to combine.

Pour the dressing over the vegetable and rice mixture to combine, then toss through the cashews and sunflower seeds. Set aside until required.

Heat a large non-stick heavy-based frying pan over medium–high heat and spray with olive oil. Cook the salmon, skin-side down, for 2–3 minutes until golden. Turn and cook for another 2 minutes for medium or continue until cooked to your liking.

Divide the salad among 4 plates or shallow bowls and top each with a piece of salmon. Scatter with sesame seeds, if using. Serve immediately, with lemon wedges alongside.

6 G FIBRE PER SERVE   GOOD SOURCE OF RESISTANT STARCH

UNITS PER SERVE ❋ BREADS AND CEREALS **1** ❋ PROTEIN **2** ❋ FRUIT **0** ❋ VEGETABLES **2** ❋ DAIRY **0** ❋ FATS AND OILS **3**

Sumac-dusted prawns *with* quinoa 'tabbouleh'

SERVES 4
PREPARATION 25 minutes
COOKING 35 minutes

800 g raw medium king prawns,
    peeled and cleaned, with tails intact
    (weight after peeling)
1½–2 teaspoons sumac
200 g green beans, trimmed
olive oil spray, for cooking
lemon wedges, to serve

QUINOA 'TABBOULEH'
¾ cup (135 g) quinoa, rinsed
2 Lebanese cucumbers,
    cut into 5 mm dice
2 roma tomatoes, cut into 5 mm dice
100 g watercress sprigs, finely chopped
100 g rocket leaves, finely chopped
small handful flat-leaf parsley leaves,
    finely chopped
small handful mint leaves,
    finely chopped
1 tablespoon extra virgin olive oil
3 teaspoons lemon juice, or to taste

To make the 'tabbouleh', add the quinoa to a large heavy-based saucepan of simmering water, reduce the heat to low and cook for 15–20 minutes until tender. Drain, rinse under cold water and drain again, then place in a large bowl and leave to cool.

Add the cucumber, tomato, watercress, rocket, parsley and mint to the quinoa and stir gently to combine, then season to taste with freshly ground black pepper. Mix the olive oil and lemon juice in a small bowl and set aside.

Meanwhile, place the prawns in a bowl, sprinkle with the sumac and season to taste with freshly ground black pepper.

Cook the beans in a saucepan of simmering water for 4 minutes or until tender but crisp. Drain and set aside.

Heat a chargrill pan over medium–high heat and spray with olive oil. Working in batches, chargrill the prawns for 2–3 minutes on each side until charred and cooked through.

Add the dressing to the 'tabbouleh' and toss to mix. Divide the 'tabbouleh' among 4 plates or shallow bowls, then top with one-quarter of the chargrilled prawns and beans. Serve with lemon wedges to the side.

8 G FIBRE PER SERVE   **LOW FODMAP**   **GOOD SOURCE OF RESISTANT STARCH**

UNITS PER SERVE ❋ BREADS AND CEREALS **1** ❋ PROTEIN **2** ❋ FRUIT **0** ❋ VEGETABLES **2.5** ❋ DAIRY **0** ❋ FATS AND OILS **1**

Cajun seafood stew

SERVES 4
PREPARATION 25 minutes
COOKING 45 minutes, plus rice cooking time

2 teaspoons garlic-infused olive oil
1 stick celery, finely chopped
1 red capsicum, seeded and
    finely chopped
1 fresh long green chilli, finely chopped
2 teaspoons sweet paprika
¼ teaspoon smoked paprika
1½ teaspoons dried
    Greek-style oregano
1½ teaspoons dried thyme
¼ teaspoon cayenne pepper
1 gluten-free, FODMAP-friendly
    chicken stock cube, dissolved in
    ½ cup (125 ml) boiling water,
    plus extra if needed
1 × 400 g tin salt-reduced
    chopped tomatoes
1 bay leaf
500 g raw medium king prawns,
    peeled and cleaned, with tails intact
    (weight after peeling)
300 g white fish fillets, skin removed,
    pin-boned and cut into
    bite-sized pieces
50 g green beans, trimmed and
    cut into 1 cm pieces
2 cups mixed salad leaves
250 g grape or cherry tomatoes, halved
1 Lebanese cucumber, halved
    lengthways and thinly sliced
    on the diagonal
½ teaspoon lemon juice
1 cup (185 g) cooked basmati rice
    (see page 41)

Heat a large heavy-based saucepan over medium heat and add the garlic oil. Add the celery and capsicum and cook for 3 minutes or until softened; add 1 tablespoon water if necessary to prevent them from sticking. Add the chilli and cook for 30 seconds or until fragrant, then add the sweet and smoked paprika, oregano, thyme and cayenne pepper and stir for 1 minute or until fragrant.

Add the stock, tomatoes and bay leaf and bring to the boil over high heat. Reduce the heat to low, then cover and cook, stirring frequently, for 25 minutes. Add the prawns, fish and green beans, pressing them gently into the sauce; add a little more stock to prevent sticking if necessary. Cover and cook for another 6–8 minutes until the prawns, fish and beans are cooked through.

Place the salad leaves, tomato and cucumber in a bowl, drizzle over the lemon juice and toss to coat.

Divide the rice among 4 plates or shallow bowls and top with one-quarter of the seafood stew, then serve with the salad to the side.

7 G FIBRE PER SERVE   LOW FODMAP

UNITS PER SERVE ❋ BREADS AND CEREALS **1** ❋ PROTEIN **2** ❋ FRUIT **0** ❋ VEGETABLES **2.5** ❋ DAIRY **0** ❋ FATS AND OILS **0.5**

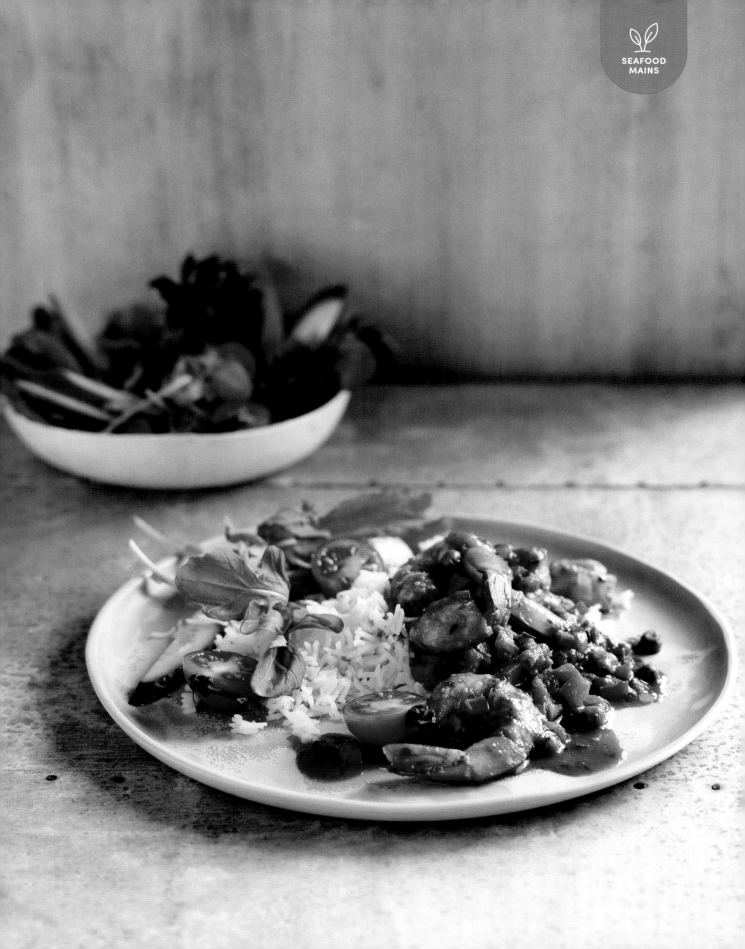

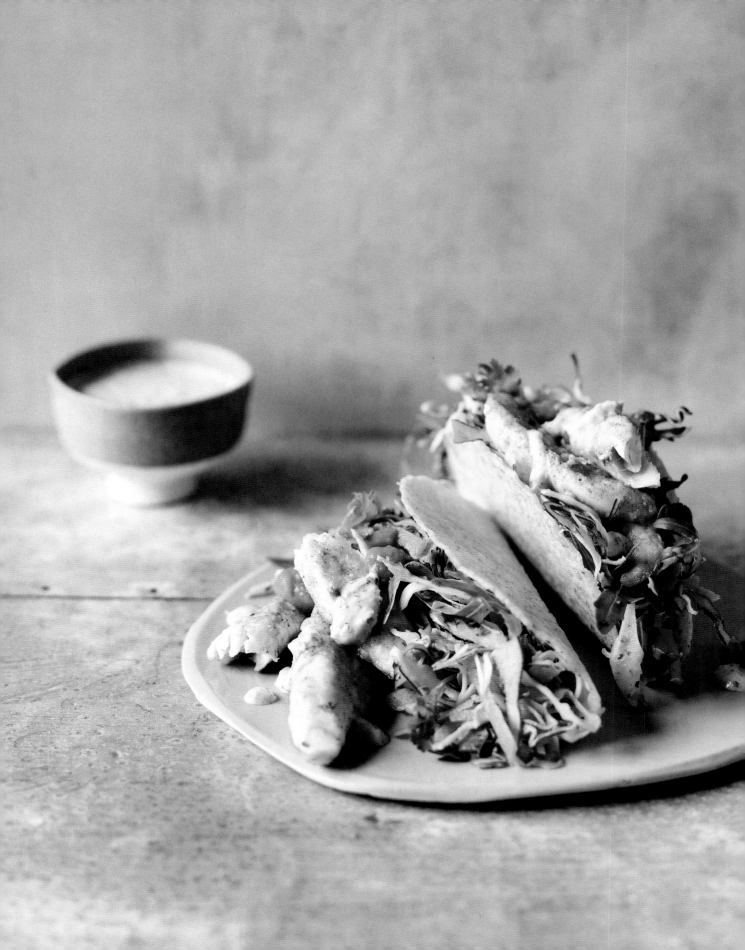

Crispy fish tacos *and* Mexican slaw

SERVES 4
PREPARATION 25 minutes
COOKING 15 minutes

4 corn taco shells
3 teaspoons spelt flour or plain flour
1 teaspoon sweet paprika
¼ teaspoon smoked paprika
600 g small flathead fillets, skin
    removed and pin-boned
olive oil spray, for cooking
200 g Refried Beans (from Breakfast
    Tortillas on page 73)

CORIANDER AND LIME
SOUR CREAM DRESSING
(MAKES ABOUT 200 ML)
2 tablespoons olive oil
5 spring onions, chopped
large handful coriander leaves
2 cloves garlic, crushed
juice of 1½ limes, or to taste
⅔ cup (160 g) light sour cream

MEXICAN SLAW
3 cups (240 g) finely shredded
    red cabbage
3 cups (240 g) finely shredded
    green cabbage
1 cup rocket leaves, trimmed
1 large carrot, coarsely grated
1 tablespoon finely chopped red onion
2 tablespoons roughly chopped
    coriander leaves

To make the dressing, place the olive oil, spring onion, coriander, garlic, lime juice and 1½ tablespoons water in a blender and blend until finely chopped. Add the sour cream and blend until a smooth puree forms. Transfer to a bowl, cover with plastic film and refrigerate until required; the dressing will thicken on chilling, but you can thin it down with a little boiling water, if desired.

To make the slaw, place all the ingredients in a bowl and toss to mix well. Set aside.

Preheat the oven to 180°C (160°C fan-forced).

Place the taco shells on a baking tray and bake according to the packet instructions.

Place the flour and paprika in a wide, shallow bowl, then season with freshly ground black pepper. Dust the flathead fillets in the seasoned flour, shaking to remove the excess.

Heat a large non-stick heavy-based frying pan over medium heat, then spray with olive oil. Add the flathead fillets and pan-fry for 6 minutes on each side or until golden and just cooked through.

Add 2 tablespoons of the dressing to the slaw; thin with a little boiling water if a thinner consistency is preferred. Stir to coat well.

Place the taco shells on a chopping board, then fill each one with one-quarter of the refried beans, a large spoonful of the Mexican slaw and one-quarter of the flathead. Drizzle a little extra dressing over, then serve with the remaining slaw and dressing to the side.

11 G FIBRE PER SERVE   **GOOD SOURCE OF RESISTANT STARCH**

UNITS PER SERVE ❋ BREADS AND CEREALS **1** ❋ PROTEIN **2** ❋ FRUIT **0** ❋ VEGETABLES **2** ❋ DAIRY **1** ❋ FATS AND OILS **2**

Prawn, zucchini, feta *and* orzo bake

SERVES 4
PREPARATION 25 minutes, plus soaking time
COOKING 40 minutes

50 g orzo (risoni)
2 tablespoons currants
boiling water, for soaking
olive oil spray, for cooking
1 small onion, finely chopped
1 clove garlic, finely chopped
¼ teaspoon chilli flakes (optional)
¼ cup (60 ml) dry white wine
1 × 400 g tin salt-reduced
    chopped tomatoes
¼ teaspoon dried Greek-style oregano
2 zucchini, cut into 5 mm dice
800 g raw medium king prawns,
    peeled and cleaned, with tails intact
    (weight after peeling)
2 tablespoons roughly chopped basil
½ teaspoon ground allspice
finely grated zest of 1 lemon
2 tablespoons lemon juice
200 g salt-reduced low-fat
    feta, crumbled
3 cups mixed salad leaves
80 g baby spinach leaves, trimmed
2 teaspoons extra virgin olive oil
½ teaspoon lemon juice, extra

Cook the orzo in a saucepan of boiling water according to the packet instructions until al dente. Drain and set aside.

Meanwhile, place the currants in a small heatproof bowl, cover with boiling water and leave to stand for 10 minutes to rehydrate. Drain and set aside.

Preheat the oven to 210°C (190° fan-forced). Spray a 1.5 litre baking dish with olive oil.

Heat a non-stick heavy-based frying pan over medium heat and spray with olive oil. Add the onion and cook for 3–4 minutes until softened and translucent, then add the garlic and chilli, if using, and cook for 30 seconds or until fragrant. Stir in the wine, then increase the heat to high and simmer for 4 minutes or until reduced by half. Add the tomatoes and oregano and stir to combine, then bring to a simmer and cook over medium heat for 5 minutes or until the sauce has thickened. Stir in the zucchini, orzo and currants, then transfer to the oiled baking dish.

Place the prawns in a bowl, add the basil, allspice, lemon zest and lemon juice and season with freshly ground black pepper. Stir to coat, then place the prawns on top of the orzo mixture. Scatter with the crumbled feta and bake for 12–15 minutes until the prawns are cooked and the feta is golden.

Meanwhile, place the salad leaves and spinach in a bowl, drizzle over the olive oil and extra lemon juice and gently toss to coat.

Divide the prawn and orzo bake among 4 plates or bowls and serve with the salad alongside.

6 G FIBRE PER SERVE

UNITS PER SERVE ❋ BREADS AND CEREALS **1** ❋ PROTEIN **2** ❋ FRUIT **0** ❋ VEGETABLES **2** ❋ DAIRY **1** ❋ FATS AND OILS **0.5**

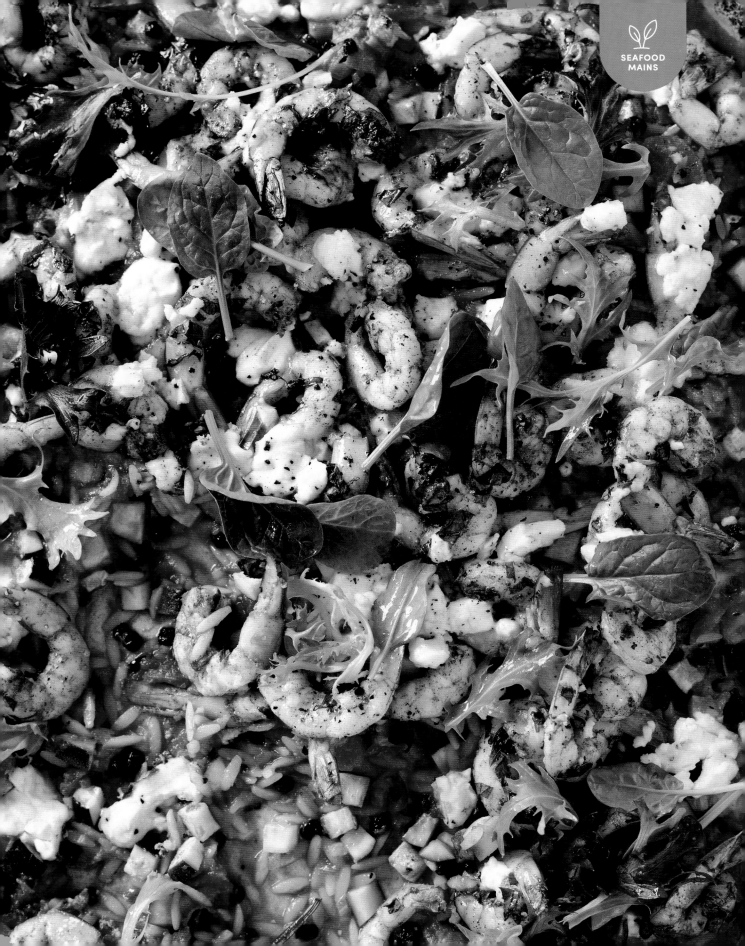

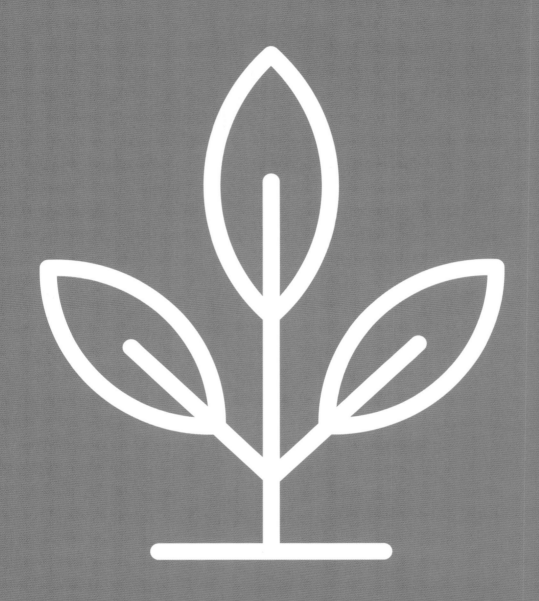

Chicken and Pork Mains

Crumbed chicken *with* potato wedges *and* fennel slaw

SERVES 4
PREPARATION 30 minutes
COOKING 45 minutes, plus potato cooking time

2 large desiree potatoes (about 300 g), cut into wedges, steamed and chilled overnight (see page 41)
olive oil spray, for cooking
½ cup (100 g) polenta
⅓ cup (55 g) LSA
¼ cup (20 g) natural (raw) rolled oats
1 egg
1 tablespoon skim milk
800 g chicken tenderloins

FENNEL SLAW
1 bulb baby fennel, trimmed and finely shaved
4 cups (320 g) finely shredded green cabbage
1 cup rocket leaves, trimmed
1 green apple, cored and cut into thin matchsticks
2 spring onions, finely chopped
1 teaspoon wholegrain mustard
1½ teaspoons white balsamic vinegar
2 teaspoons extra virgin olive oil
2 tablespoons raw cashews, roasted and roughly chopped

Preheat the oven to 200°C (180°C fan-forced). Line 2 baking trays with baking paper.

Place the potato wedges on a lined baking tray, spray with olive oil and roast for 25 minutes, then turn and roast for another 20 minutes or until golden and crisp.

Meanwhile, place the polenta, LSA and oats in a shallow, wide bowl and stir to combine. Place the egg and milk in another shallow, wide bowl and whisk until lightly beaten. Working in batches, dip the chicken into the egg mixture to coat, drain off the excess, then dust with the polenta mixture. Press the polenta mixture on firmly to coat well. Place on the other lined tray and refrigerate until ready to cook.

To make the slaw, place the fennel, cabbage, rocket, apple and spring onion in a bowl and toss to combine. Combine the mustard and vinegar in a small bowl, then stir in the olive oil until emulsified. Season to taste with freshly ground black pepper, then set aside.

Heat a large non-stick heavy-based frying pan over low–medium heat and spray with olive oil. Spray the chicken with olive oil, then add to the pan and cook for 5–6 minutes on each side until golden and cooked through; reduce the temperature if necessary as the chicken needs to cook through without the coating burning.

Add the dressing to the slaw and toss to coat, then scatter over the cashews. Divide the chicken, wedges and slaw among 4 plates and serve immediately.

10 G FIBRE PER SERVE   GOOD SOURCE OF RESISTANT STARCH

UNITS PER SERVE   ❀ BREADS AND CEREALS **1** ❀ PROTEIN **2** ❀ FRUIT **0** ❀ VEGETABLES **2** ❀ DAIRY **0** ❀ FATS AND OILS **3**

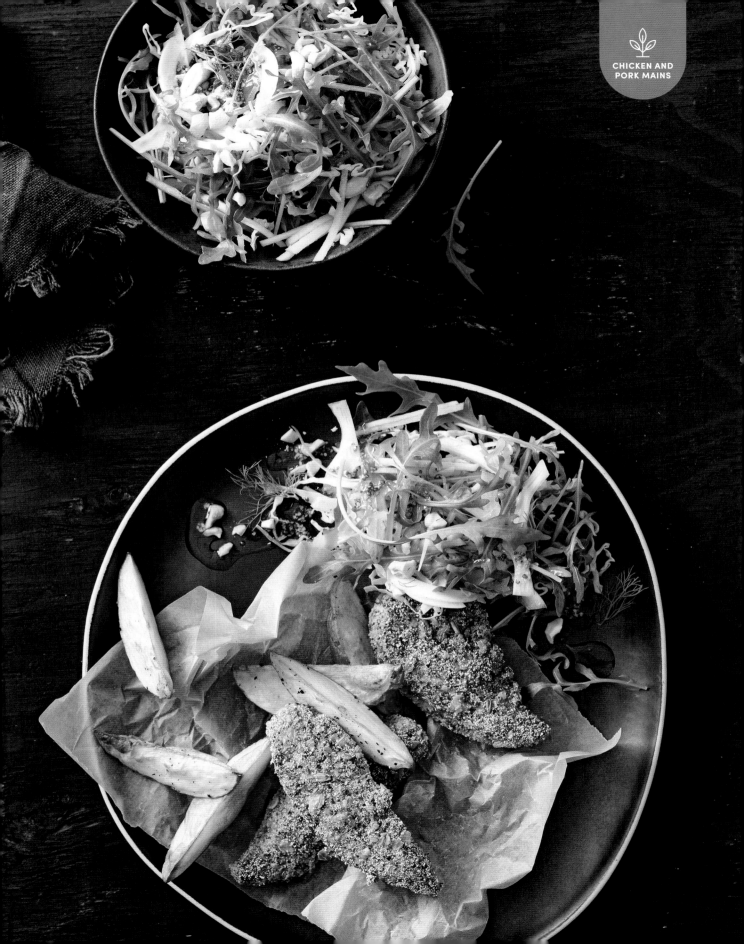

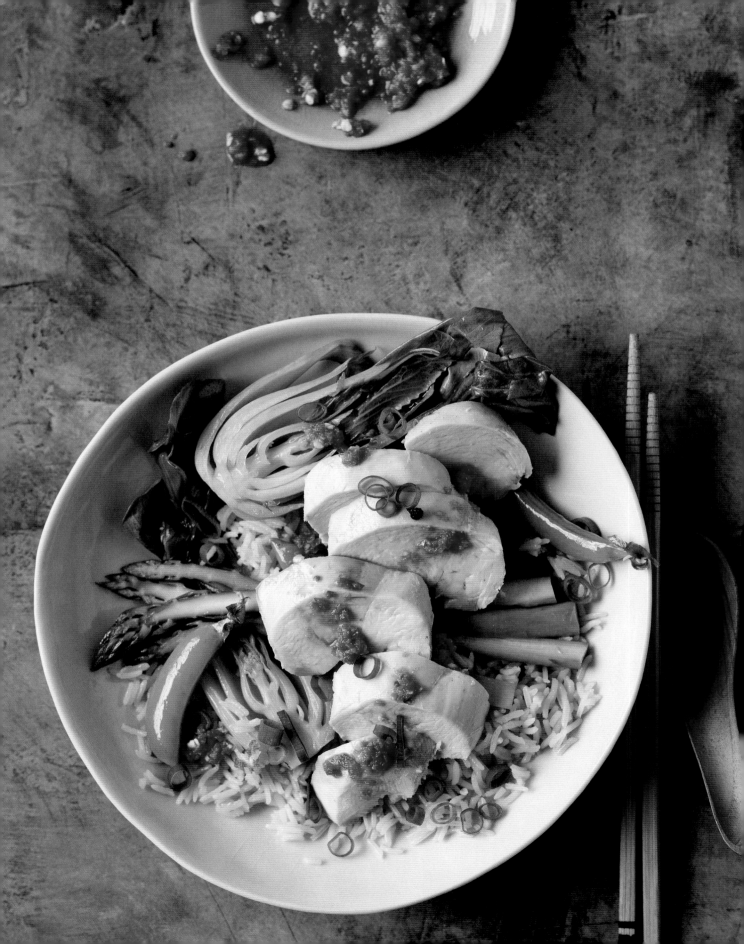

Hainan-style chicken *and* ginger rice *with* Asian greens *and* chilli dipping sauce

SERVES 4
PREPARATION 20 minutes, plus standing time
COOKING 45 minutes

4 × 200 g chicken breast fillets
1 litre salt-reduced chicken stock
4 spring onions, white parts only
    (reserve green tops, finely
    chopped, to serve)
4 thin slices ginger, plus
    ½ teaspoon finely grated ginger
1 star anise
1 teaspoon Sichuan pepper
olive oil spray, for cooking
½ cup (100 g) basmati rice
2 baby bok choy, trimmed and
    halved or quartered lengthways
1 bunch asparagus, bases trimmed,
    cut into 5 cm lengths
100 g sugar snap peas, trimmed

CHILLI DIPPING SAUCE
2 fresh long red chillies, seeded
    and roughly chopped (optional)
½ small clove garlic, crushed
1 teaspoon finely grated ginger
3 teaspoons lime juice, or to taste
1 teaspoon pure maple syrup

Place the chicken, stock, spring onion, sliced ginger, star anise and Sichuan pepper in a deep heavy-based frying pan with a lid and bring to a simmer over high heat. Reduce the heat to low and simmer for 15–20 minutes until the chicken is cooked through. Remove from the heat and leave to stand, covered, for 10 minutes. Transfer the chicken to a plate, cover loosely with foil and keep warm. Strain the stock and reserve.

Meanwhile, to make the dipping sauce, place all the ingredients in a small food processor and pulse to form a smooth paste. Transfer to a bowl and set aside.

Heat a heavy-based saucepan over medium heat, then spray with olive oil. Add the grated ginger and rice and stir for 1 minute or until fragrant. Measure ¾ cup (180 ml) of the reserved stock and add to the pan. Bring to the boil over high heat, then reduce the heat to low, cover and cook for 12 minutes or until all the stock has been absorbed and the rice is tender. Leave to stand, covered, for 5 minutes.

Pour the remaining stock into a clean saucepan and bring to the boil.

Working in batches, steam the bok choy, asparagus and sugar snap peas for 2–3 minutes until tender but crisp.

Add the chicken breasts to the hot stock to warm through, if necessary. Remove and cut into thick slices on the diagonal. Divide the rice among 4 shallow bowls, then serve a sliced chicken breast on top of each, along with the steamed vegetables. Serve with the bowl of dipping sauce to the side.

4 G FIBRE PER SERVE

UNITS PER SERVE ✽ BREADS AND CEREALS **2** ✽ PROTEIN **2** ✽ FRUIT **0** ✽ VEGETABLES **1.5** ✽ DAIRY **0** ✽ FATS AND OILS **0**

Cheat's chicken paella

SERVES 4
PREPARATION 20 minutes, plus standing time
COOKING 45 minutes, plus rice cooking time

olive oil spray, for cooking
600 g chicken breast or thigh fillets,
    cut into bite-sized pieces
1 red onion, finely chopped
1 large red capsicum, seeded, ½ finely
    chopped and ½ thinly sliced
1 clove garlic, chopped
1 teaspoon sweet paprika
1½ cups (375 ml) salt-reduced
    tomato passata
pinch of saffron threads, soaked
    in 2 tablespoons boiling water
    for 10 minutes
150 g broad beans
1½ cups (180 g) frozen peas
150 g green beans, trimmed
1 cup (185 g) cooked basmati rice
    (see page 41)
2 cups mixed salad leaves
lemon wedges, to serve

Heat a heavy-based frying pan with a lid over medium heat and spray with olive oil. Add the chicken and cook, stirring for 4–5 minutes until browned all over. Transfer to a bowl and set aside.

Spray the pan with a little more olive oil, then add the onion, chopped capsicum and garlic and cook, stirring occasionally, for 5 minutes or until softened. Stir in the paprika and cook for 30 seconds. Add the passata and bring to a simmer. Stir in the saffron mixture, chicken and ½ cup (125 ml) water and bring to the boil over high heat. Cover, reduce the heat to low and cook for 20–25 minutes until the chicken is cooked through.

Preheat the oven grill to high. Line a baking tray with foil, top with the sliced capsicum and grill for 5 minutes or until softened and the skin is slightly charred.

Cook the broad beans in a small saucepan of simmering water for 3 minutes, then remove with a slotted spoon, run under cold water and double-peel. Add the peas to the pan of simmering water and cook for 3 minutes or until tender. Drain. Cook the beans in a saucepan of simmering water for 4 minutes or until tender but a little crisp. Add the capsicum, broad beans, peas and beans to the chicken mixture.

Divide the rice among 4 plates or bowls, top each bowl with one-quarter of the chicken and vegetable mixture and serve immediately with the salad leaves and lemon wedges to the side.

11 G FIBRE PER SERVE   GOOD SOURCE OF RESISTANT STARCH

UNITS PER SERVE ❋ BREADS AND CEREALS **1** ❋ PROTEIN **2** ❋ FRUIT **0** ❋ VEGETABLES **2** ❋ DAIRY **0** ❋ FATS AND OILS **0**

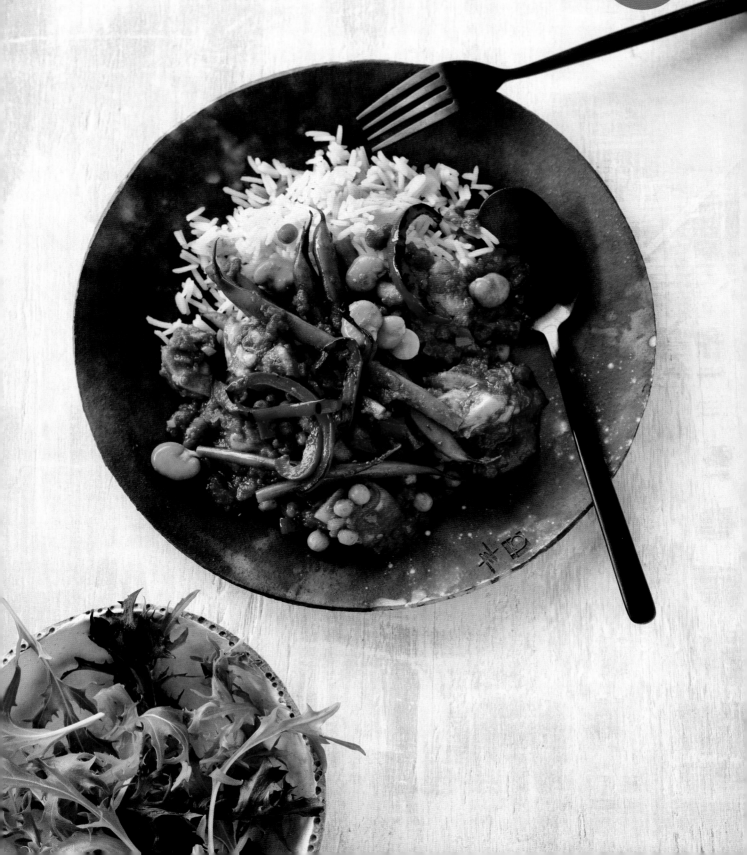

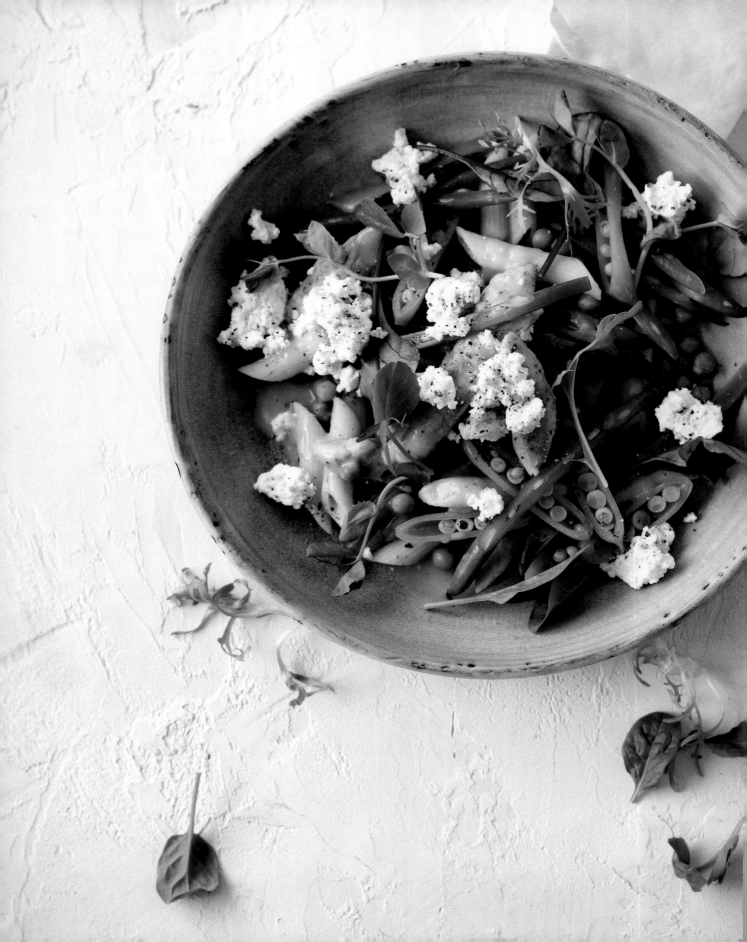

Pasta *with* chicken, cannellini bean puree, peas *and* beans

SERVES 4
PREPARATION 20 minutes
COOKING 25 minutes

⅔ cup (70 g) penne rigate,
  conchiglie or fusilli
olive oil spray, for cooking
1 cup (120 g) frozen peas
150 g sugar snap peas
150 g green beans, halved
  on the diagonal
400 g chicken tenderloins, thinly sliced
juice of ½ lemon
3 sprigs thyme, leaves picked and
  finely chopped
150 g reduced-fat ricotta
2 cups mixed salad leaves

CANNELLINI BEAN PUREE
1 × 400 g tin salt-reduced cannellini
  beans, drained and rinsed
¾ cup (180 ml) salt-reduced chicken
  or vegetable stock
1 clove garlic, crushed
1 teaspoon finely grated lemon zest
lemon juice, to taste

To make the puree, place the cannellini beans, stock, garlic and ¼ cup (60 ml) water in a small heavy-based saucepan, bring to the boil over high heat and cook for 10 minutes to warm the beans through. Drain the beans, reserving the stock, and transfer to a blender or food processor. Add the lemon zest and 2 tablespoons of the reserved stock and process or blend to a puree, adding a little extra stock if a thinner consistency is desired. Reserve any remaining stock. Return the puree to the saucepan, stir in lemon juice to taste and keep warm.

Meanwhile, cook the pasta in a large saucepan of simmering water according to the packet instructions until al dente. Drain, reserving ¼ cup (60 ml) of the pasta water and set aside. Cook the peas in a saucepan of simmering water for 3 minutes or until tender. Drain and set aside. Cook the sugar snap peas and beans in a saucepan of simmering water for 2 minutes or until tender but crisp. Drain and set aside with the peas.

Heat a large non-stick heavy-based frying pan over medium heat and spray with olive oil. Add the chicken and cook, stirring constantly, for 5–6 minutes until cooked through. Squeeze in the lemon juice and stir in the thyme. Add the pasta, half the remaining stock and half of the cannellini bean puree to the pan, stir to combine and season to taste with freshly ground black pepper. Add a little of the reserved pasta cooking water if a thinner sauce is preferred. Gently stir in the peas, sugar snap peas and beans. (Leftover cannellini bean puree can be stored in an airtight container in the refrigerator for up to 3 days.)

Divide the pasta mixture among 4 bowls, crumble one-quarter of the ricotta over each and serve with the salad leaves alongside.

11 G FIBRE PER SERVE **GOOD SOURCE OF RESISTANT STARCH**

UNITS PER SERVE ✿ BREADS AND CEREALS **1** ✿ PROTEIN **2** ✿ FRUIT **0** ✿ VEGETABLES **2** ✿ DAIRY **0.5** ✿ FATS AND OILS **0**

Sweet *and* sour chicken stir-fry

SERVES 4
PREPARATION 20 minutes
COOKING 10 minutes

2 tablespoons garlic-infused olive oil
800 g chicken tenderloins,
    halved on the diagonal
3 cm piece ginger, finely grated
2 sticks celery, sliced on the diagonal
4 zucchini, halved lengthways, sliced
    on the diagonal
200 g peeled, cored pineapple,
    chopped
finely grated zest and juice of
    1 small lemon
1 tablespoon tamari (gluten-free
    soy sauce)
6 baby bok choy, leaves separated

Heat the olive oil in a large wok over high heat. Add the chicken and ginger and stir-fry for 4 minutes or until the chicken is tender and caramelised.

Add all the remaining ingredients and 2 tablespoons water. Stir-fry for 2 minutes or until the vegetables are just tender and the greens are just starting to wilt. Divide evenly among 4 plates and serve.

If desired, you can serve this stir-fry with 2 cups (370 g) of cooked brown basmati rice (see page 41; this will add 1 unit of breads and cereals and 3 g fibre per serve).

4 G FIBRE PER SERVE   **LOW FODMAP**

UNITS PER SERVE ❋ BREADS AND CEREALS **1** ❋ PROTEIN **2** ❋ FRUIT **0.5** ❋ VEGETABLES **2** ❋ DAIRY **0** ❋ FATS AND OILS **2**

Chicken fajita *and* avocado bowls

SERVES 4
PREPARATION 20 minutes, plus refrigerating time
COOKING 25 minutes

---

800 g chicken tenderloins, thinly sliced
2 teaspoons sweet paprika
1½ teaspoons dried
    Greek-style oregano
¼ teaspoon ground cinnamon
juice of 1 lime
handful coriander leaves,
    roughly chopped
small handful flat-leaf parsley leaves,
    roughly chopped
1 clove garlic, crushed
½ teaspoon ground cumin
2 teaspoons extra virgin olive oil
½ cup (125 g) light sour cream
olive oil spray, for cooking
8 hard taco shells
100 g reduced-fat cheddar,
    coarsely grated
2 tomatoes, halved and thinly sliced
200 g mixed salad leaves, washed
    and dried
160 g avocado, cut into 1 cm dice

Place the chicken in a bowl, add the paprika, oregano, cinnamon and half of the lime juice and stir to mix well. Season with freshly ground black pepper.

Place the coriander, parsley, garlic, cumin and remaining lime juice in a small food processor or blender and process until finely chopped. Remove 2 tablespoons of the paste and mix with the olive oil, then add to the chicken and stir to coat. Cover with plastic film and refrigerate.

Transfer the remaining coriander paste to a small bowl and stir in the sour cream. Cover with plastic film and refrigerate until needed.

Heat a large non-stick heavy-based frying pan over medium heat and spray with olive oil. Working in 4 batches so as not to crowd the pan, stir-fry the chicken for 5–6 minutes until golden and cooked through, transferring each batch to a bowl while you cook the remaining chicken.

Divide the taco shells evenly among 4 plates, then add one-quarter of the chicken, cheese, tomato, lettuce and avocado to each one and serve with the coriander cream sauce to the side.

8 G FIBRE PER SERVE

UNITS PER SERVE ❋ BREADS AND CEREALS **1** ❋ PROTEIN **2** ❋ FRUIT **0** ❋ VEGETABLES **2** ❋ DAIRY **1** ❋ FATS AND OILS **2**

Antipasto barbecue chicken

SERVES 4
PREPARATION 20 minutes
COOKING 10 minutes, plus standing time

2 tablespoons garlic-infused olive oil
2 teaspoons mixed dried herbs
800 g chicken breast fillet, cut on
   the diagonal into thick slices
1 eggplant, sliced into rounds
4 zucchini, sliced on the diagonal
4 roma tomatoes, halved lengthways
¼ cup (60 ml) balsamic vinegar
100 g pitted kalamata olives
100 g salt-reduced Greek feta,
   crumbled
1 small bunch flat-leaf parsley, leaves
   picked, stems finely chopped

Preheat a barbecue chargrill plate and flat plate to high heat.

Place the olive oil, herbs, chicken, eggplant, zucchini and tomato in a large bowl and toss until well coated. Using tongs, transfer the chicken to the barbecue chargrill plate and the vegetable mixture to the flat plate. Cook, turning the vegetables occasionally and the chicken only once, for 10 minutes or until the chicken is golden and cooked through. Transfer the chicken and vegetables to a large bowl, cover loosely with foil and rest for 3 minutes.

Add the remaining ingredients to the chicken mixture and toss gently to combine. Season to taste with freshly ground black pepper and serve immediately.

If desired, you can serve this meal with 2 cups (370 g) of cooked quinoa (this will add 1 unit of breads and cereals and 3 g fibre per serve).

9 G FIBRE PER SERVE   LOW FODMAP

UNITS PER SERVE ❀ BREADS AND CEREALS **0** ❀ PROTEIN **2** ❀ FRUIT **0** ❀ VEGETABLES **2.5** ❀ DAIRY **1** ❀ FATS AND OILS **3.5**

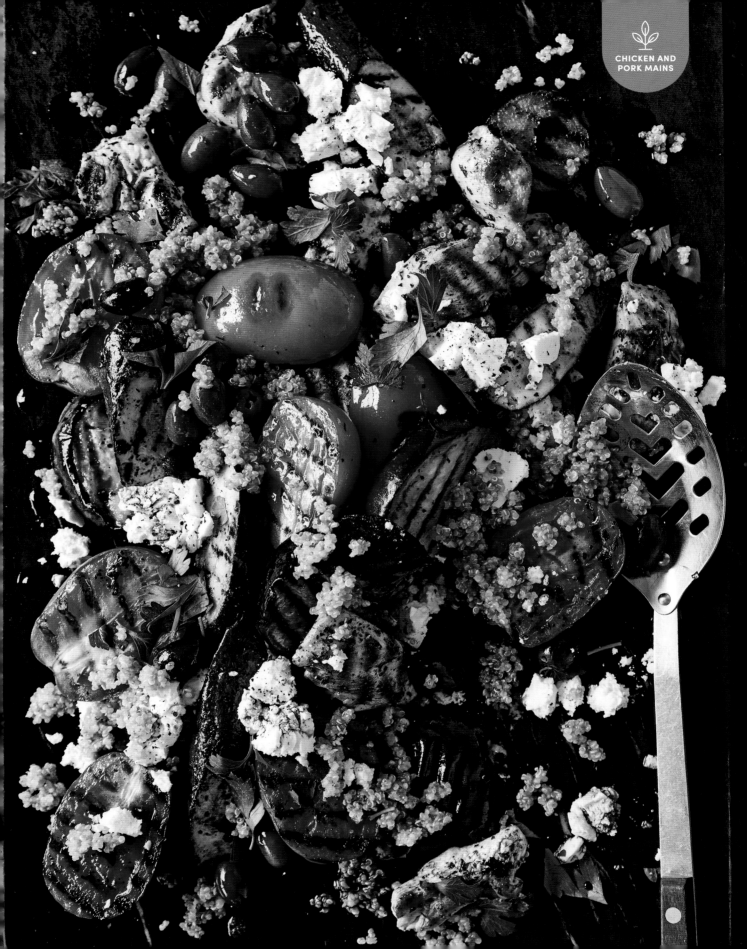

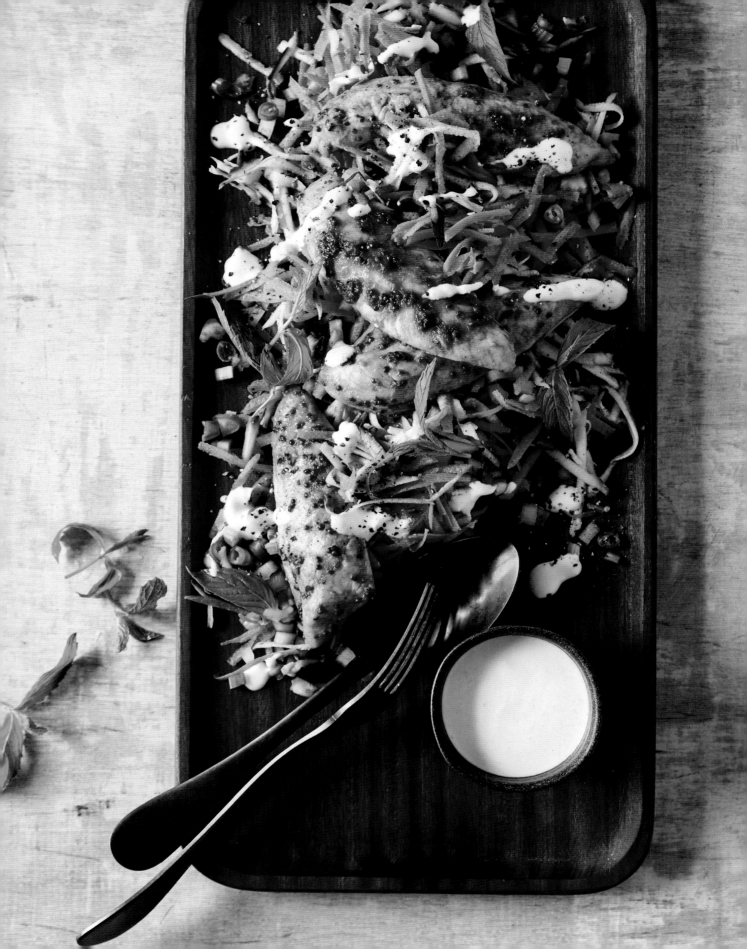

Grilled turmeric tenderloins
with Indian slaw

SERVES 4
PREPARATION 25 minutes
COOKING 15 minutes, plus standing time

---

800 g chicken tenderloins
2 tablespoons garlic-infused olive oil
2 teaspoons ground turmeric
1 tablespoon wholegrain mustard
2 teaspoons pure maple syrup
    (optional)

INDIAN SLAW
¾ cup (210 g) lactose-free
    natural yoghurt
3 cm piece ginger, finely grated
finely grated zest and juice of
    1 small lemon
2 sticks celery, cut into thin matchsticks
2 carrots, coarsely grated
100 g green beans, thinly sliced
    into rounds
4 zucchini, coarsely grated
1 cup small mint leaves

Preheat the oven grill to high and line a large baking tray with foil.

Place the chicken, olive oil, turmeric, mustard and maple syrup (if using) in a large bowl and toss until the chicken is well coated. Season to taste with freshly ground black pepper. Transfer to the prepared tray and cook under the grill, turning once, for 12–15 minutes until the chicken is golden and cooked through. Transfer to a chopping board, cover loosely with foil and rest for 3 minutes, then cut on the diagonal into thick slices.

Meanwhile, to make the Indian slaw, whisk together the yoghurt, ginger, lemon zest and juice in a large bowl. Season to taste with freshly ground black pepper. Add the remaining ingredients and toss well to combine.

Divide the chicken evenly among 4 plates and serve with the Indian slaw.

You can marinate the chicken mixture for up to 2 days. Just cover it tightly and keep it chilled.

If desired, you can serve this meal with 2 cups (370 g) of cooked brown basmati rice (see page 41; this will add 1 unit of breads and cereals and 3 g fibre per serve).

6 G FIBRE PER SERVE   **LOW FODMAP**

UNITS PER SERVE   ✳ BREADS AND CEREALS **0**   ✳ PROTEIN **2**   ✳ FRUIT **0**   ✳ VEGETABLES **2**   ✳ DAIRY **1**   ✳ FATS AND OILS **2**

Five-spice braised pork *with* Asian greens, beans *and* rice

SERVES 4
PREPARATION 25 minutes, plus standing time
COOKING 1 hour

The protein in this recipe comes from the legumes and the meat.

3 teaspoons garlic-infused olive oil
600 g pork tenderloin, all visible fat removed, cut into 2 cm cubes
1.5 cm piece ginger, finely grated
¼ teaspoon five-spice powder, or to taste
1 tablespoon tamari (gluten-free soy sauce)
1 teaspoon white balsamic vinegar
1 star anise
4 gluten-free, FODMAP-friendly chicken stock cubes dissolved in 2½ cups (625 ml) boiling water
2 teaspoons hoisin sauce
1 bunch choy sum, trimmed and cut into 4 cm lengths
1 bunch gai lan, trimmed and cut into 4 cm lengths
250 g green beans, halved on the diagonal

BEANS AND RICE
1 teaspoon garlic-infused olive oil
1 stick celery, finely chopped
½ cup (100 g) basmati rice
200 g tinned salt-reduced kidney beans, drained and rinsed
⅔ cup (50 g) baby spinach leaves

Heat the olive oil in an enamelled cast-iron casserole dish or heavy-based saucepan over medium heat. Working in batches, if necessary, add the pork and cook, stirring for 4–5 minutes until lightly browned. Transfer to a bowl and set aside.

Add the ginger and five-spice powder and cook, stirring, for 1 minute or until fragrant. Return the pork to the pan, season well with freshly ground black pepper and stir to coat in the five-spice mixture. Add the tamari, vinegar, star anise and stock. Bring to a simmer, then reduce the heat to low and simmer, covered and stirring occasionally, for 20 minutes then uncover and simmer for a further 15 minutes or until the pork is tender.

Meanwhile, to make the beans and rice, heat a heavy-based saucepan over medium heat and add the olive oil. Add the celery and cook for 3 minutes or until softened. Stir in the rice, then add ¾ cup (180 ml) water and bring to the boil over high heat. Cover, reduce the heat to low and cook for 12 minutes or until the water has been absorbed and the rice is tender. Stir in the kidney beans and spinach, then cover and leave to stand for 10 minutes.

Stir the hoisin sauce into the braised pork mixture and simmer for 1 minute. Add the choy sum, gai lan, and beans, then cover and cook over medium heat for 3 minutes or until the vegetables are tender but still crisp and the sauce is thickened.

Divide the beans and rice among 4 bowls or plates, top each bowl with one-quarter of the braised pork and vegetables, then serve.

9 G FIBRE PER SERVE

UNITS PER SERVE ❋ BREADS AND CEREALS **1** ❋ PROTEIN **2** ❋ FRUIT **0** ❋ VEGETABLES **2** ❋ DAIRY **0** ❋ FATS AND OILS **2**

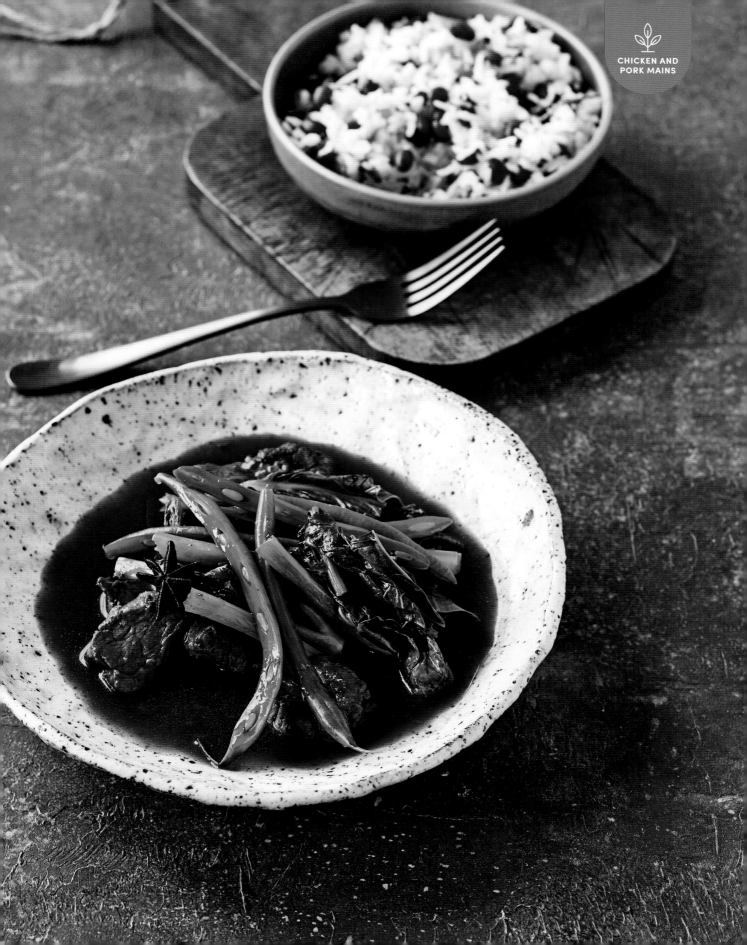

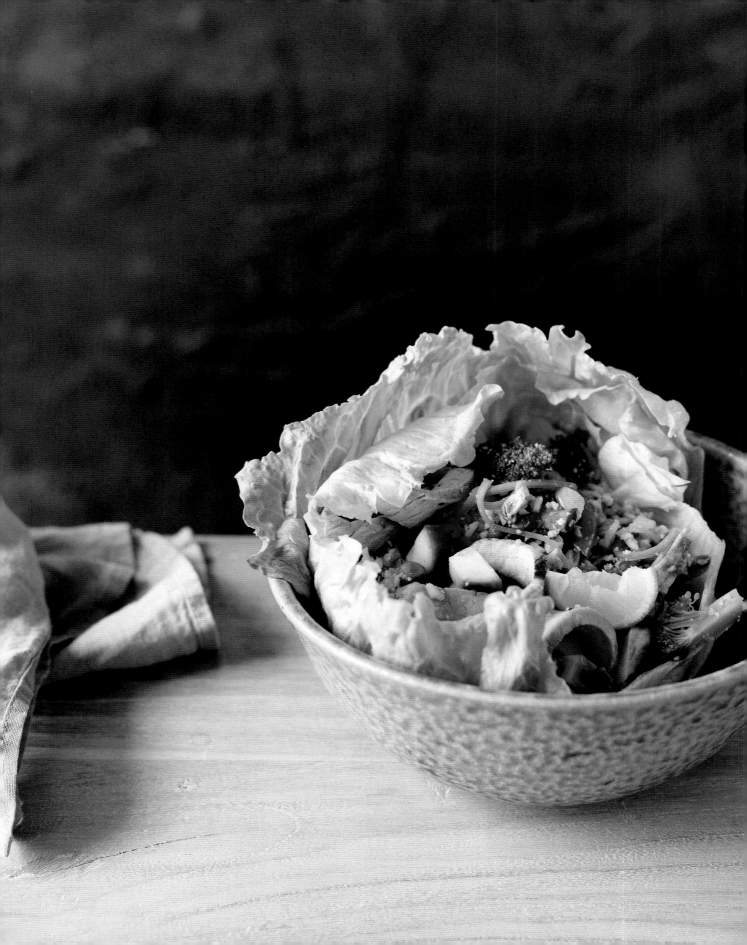

Lemongrass pork *with* cauliflower fried rice *and* cashews

SERVES 4
PREPARATION 25 minutes
COOKING 25 minutes, plus rice cooking time

3 teaspoons fish sauce

2 cloves garlic, finely chopped

2 stalks lemongrass, white part only, finely chopped

1 teaspoon freshly ground white pepper

4 × 200 g pork butterfly (loin medallion) steaks, all visible fat removed

olive oil spray, for cooking

8 inner iceberg lettuce leaf cups

1 Lebanese cucumber, chopped

⅓ cup (50 g) roasted unsalted cashews, coarsely chopped

lime wedges, to serve

CAULIFLOWER FRIED RICE

500 g cauliflower, cut into small florets

1½ cups (180 g) frozen peas

olive oil spray, for cooking

150 g sugar snap peas, trimmed

120 g snake beans, cut into 3 cm lengths

1 small head broccoli, trimmed and cut into small florets

120 g button mushrooms, trimmed and thickly sliced

4 spring onions, finely chopped

1 carrot, coarsely grated

1 cup (185 g) cooked basmati rice (see page 41)

2 teaspoons salt-reduced soy sauce

sesame oil, for drizzling

Place the fish sauce, garlic, lemongrass and pepper in a small bowl and stir to combine. Place the pork in a baking dish, spoon the marinade over to coat each side, cover and set aside.

To make the fried rice, place the cauliflower in a food processor and process until finely chopped, then set aside. Cook the peas in a saucepan of simmering water for 3 minutes until tender, then drain and set aside.

Spray a chargrill pan with olive oil and heat over high heat (or heat a barbecue grill plate to high). Add the pork and cook for 5–6 minutes on each side until browned and just cooked through. Transfer to a plate and cover loosely with foil to rest.

Spray a wok or large non-stick heavy-based frying pan with olive oil and heat over medium heat. Add the sugar snap peas and beans and stir-fry for 2–3 minutes until just softened. Transfer to a heatproof bowl and set aside. Add the broccoli and mushrooms to the wok, spray with more oil if necessary, and stir-fry for 3 minutes or until tender, then transfer to the bowl. Add the cauliflower, spring onion and carrot to the wok and stir-fry for 2 minutes, then add the rice, peas, reserved vegetables and soy sauce and stir-fry for 2–3 minutes until heated through. Drizzle with sesame oil and set aside.

Cut the pork into thick slices on the diagonal. Place two lettuce cups into the base of 4 bowls. Add one-quarter of the fried rice and cucumber and a sliced pork steak to each one. Scatter over the chopped cashews and serve immediately with lime wedges.

15 G FIBRE PER SERVE   GOOD SOURCE OF RESISTANT STARCH

UNITS PER SERVE ❀ BREADS AND CEREALS **1** ❀ PROTEIN **2** ❀ FRUIT **0** ❀ VEGETABLES **3.5** ❀ DAIRY **0** ❀ FATS AND OILS **2**

Fast pork chilli *with* red rice *and* beans

SERVES 4
PREPARATION 25 minutes, plus standing time
COOKING 30 minutes

3 tomatoes, seeded and finely chopped
2 tablespoons lime juice
1 teaspoon chilli powder
1 teaspoon ground cumin
½ teaspoon ground allspice
olive oil spray, for cooking
1 small red onion, halved lengthways
    and thinly sliced
2 cloves garlic, finely chopped
1 × 600 g pork fillet, all visible fat
    removed, thinly sliced
2 cups mixed salad leaves
lime wedges, to serve

RED RICE AND BEANS
olive oil spray, for cooking
1 small onion, finely chopped
1 clove garlic, finely chopped
½ cup (100 g) basmati rice
50 g salt-reduced tomato paste
¾ cup (180 ml) salt-reduced chicken
    stock or water
200 g salt-reduced kidney beans,
    drained and rinsed

GUACAMOLE SALAD
80 g avocado, cut into 1.5 cm dice
250 g grape tomatoes, halved
1 tablespoon finely chopped red onion
½ small clove garlic, finely chopped
juice of 1 lime
lime halves and coriander sprigs,
    to serve

To make the red rice and beans, heat a heavy-based saucepan over medium heat and spray with olive oil. Add the onion and cook for 3 minutes or until softened, then add the garlic and cook for 30 seconds or until fragrant. Stir in the rice to coat with the onion mixture, then stir in the tomato paste. Add the stock or water and bring to the boil over high heat. Reduce the heat to low, then cover and cook for 12 minutes or until all the liquid has been absorbed and the rice is tender. Stir in the kidney beans, then cover and cook for another 2 minutes or until heated through. Gently fluff with a fork, cover, and leave to stand for 10 minutes before serving.

To make the guacamole salad, place the avocado, tomato and onion in a bowl and gently stir to mix. Add the garlic to the lime juice, then add to the salad and stir gently to mix through. Just before serving, gently stir through the coriander leaves.

Meanwhile, mix the tomato, lime juice, chilli powder, cumin and allspice in a small bowl. Heat a large heavy-based frying pan or wok over high heat, then spray with olive oil. Add the onion and cook for 3 minutes or until softened, then add the garlic and cook for 30 seconds or until fragrant. Spray with a little more oil, if necessary, then add the pork, in batches if necessary, and stir-fry for 5–6 minutes until golden and cooked through. Add the tomato mixture and stir to mix well, then cook for 3–4 minutes until heated through.

Divide the red rice and beans among 4 bowls, then top each bowl with one-quarter of the pork. Serve the guacamole salad, lime halves and coriander alongside.

11 G FIBRE PER SERVE

UNITS PER SERVE ❁ BREADS AND CEREALS **1** ❁ PROTEIN **2** ❁ FRUIT **0** ❁ VEGETABLES **2** ❁ DAIRY **0** ❁ FATS AND OILS **2**

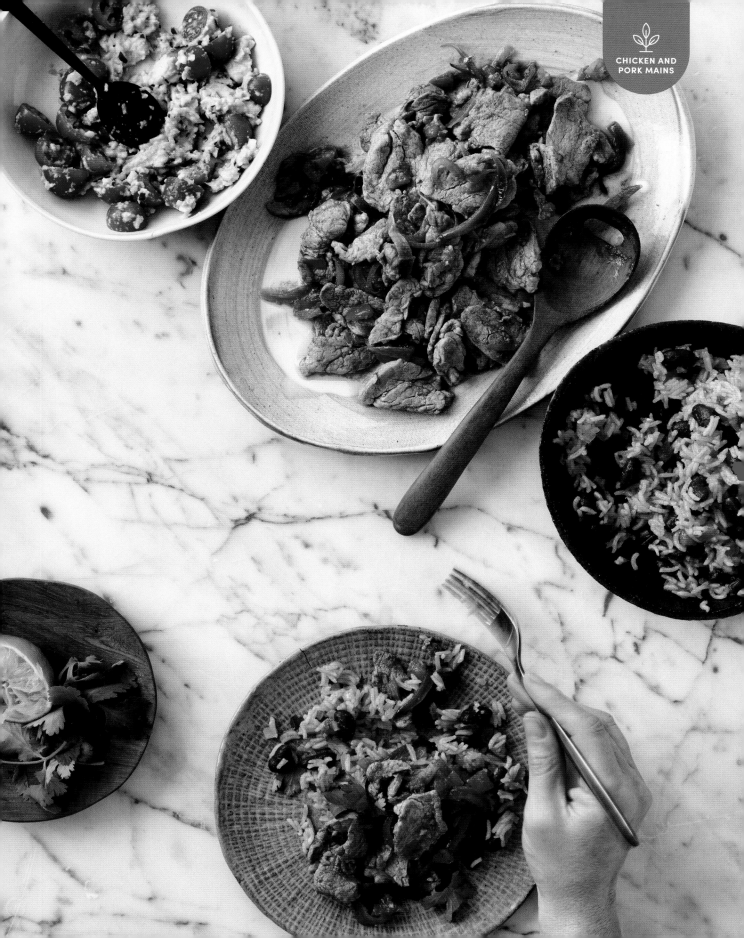

Rosemary *and* thyme pork steaks *with* Russian potato salad

SERVES 4
PREPARATION 25 minutes, plus standing time
COOKING 20 minutes, plus potato cooking time

2 long sprigs rosemary, leaves picked
   and finely chopped
2 teaspoons finely chopped thyme
finely grated zest of 1 lemon
4 × 200 g pork butterfly (loin medallion)
   steaks, all visible fat removed
olive oil spray, for cooking
2 bunches broccolini, bases trimmed
2 bunches asparagus, bases trimmed

RUSSIAN POTATO SALAD
600 g desiree or Nicola potatoes,
   halved, steamed, drizzled with a
   little vinegar and chilled overnight,
   then cut into 1 cm dice (see page 41)
1½ cups (180 g) frozen peas
2 dill pickles or gherkins, finely chopped
¼ small red onion, finely chopped
small handful flat-leaf parsley leaves,
   roughly chopped
2 teaspoons apple cider vinegar, plus
   extra for drizzling
1 tablespoon extra virgin olive oil

Combine the rosemary, thyme and lemon zest in a small bowl. Season the pork steaks all over with freshly ground black pepper, then rub the herb mixture evenly over to coat both sides. Cover with plastic film and leave to stand while preparing the potato salad.

To make the potato salad, place the potato in a large bowl. Cook the peas in a saucepan of boiling water for 3 minutes or until tender, then drain and run under cold water to cool. Add to the bowl of potato, then add the dill pickle or gherkin, onion and parsley. Combine the vinegar and olive oil in a small bowl, then drizzle over the salad and toss gently to combine.

Heat a non-stick heavy-based frying pan over medium heat, then spray with olive oil. Add the pork steaks and cook for 5–6 minutes on each side until golden and just cooked through. Meanwhile, steam the broccolini and asparagus in a steamer basket over a saucepan of simmering water for 3 minutes or until tender but crisp.

Serve the pork steaks with the potato salad, broccolini and asparagus alongside.

10 G FIBRE PER SERVE   GOOD SOURCE OF RESISTANT STARCH

UNITS PER SERVE ❄ BREADS AND CEREALS **1** ❄ PROTEIN **2** ❄ FRUIT **0** ❄ VEGETABLES **2** ❄ DAIRY **0** ❄ FATS AND OILS **1**

Fennel-crusted pork cutlets *with* pea *and* potato mash, *and* fennel, rocket *and* apple salad

SERVES 4
PREPARATION 25 minutes, plus standing time
COOKING 15 minutes, plus potato cooking time

2 teaspoons fennel seeds
1 teaspoon coriander seeds
1 tablespoon finely chopped thyme
1 clove garlic, crushed
1 tablespoon lemon juice
4 × 200 g pork cutlets, all visible
    fat trimmed
olive oil spray, for cooking

PEA AND POTATO MASH
2 cups (240 g) frozen peas
600 g potatoes, quartered, steamed
    and chilled overnight (see page 41)
⅓ cup (80 g) light sour cream

FENNEL, ROCKET AND APPLE SALAD
2 cups rocket leaves, trimmed
1 bulb fennel, trimmed and shaved
1 small pink lady apple, cored,
    quartered and cut into 5 mm thick
    slices or thin matchsticks
2 pale inner sticks celery, thinly sliced
⅓ cup (50 g) roasted unsalted cashews
¼ cup (60 g) light sour cream
3 teaspoons lemon juice
1 tablespoon finely chopped chives

Place the fennel seeds, coriander seeds, thyme and garlic in a mortar and pound with a pestle until a paste forms. Stir in the lemon juice and season to taste with freshly ground black pepper. Place the pork cutlets in a baking dish and rub evenly with the fennel mixture to coat both sides. Cover with plastic film and leave to stand while preparing the mash.

To make the mash, cook the peas in a saucepan of simmering water for 3 minutes or until tender, then drain and set aside. Warm the potatoes in a microwave-safe container on high setting for 2 minutes or until warmed through. (Alternatively, add them to the pan of peas to warm through, then drain together.) Return the peas to the pan, add the warmed potatoes, then mash with a vegetable masher until smooth. Stir in the sour cream and season to taste with freshly ground black pepper. Cover and keep warm.

Heat a chargrill pan over high heat (or a barbecue grill plate to high) and spray with olive oil. Add the pork cutlets and cook for 4–5 minutes on each side until browned and cooked through. Transfer to a plate, cover loosely with foil and leave to rest.

Meanwhile, to make the salad, place the rocket, fennel, apple, celery and cashews in a bowl and mix to combine. Place the sour cream, lemon juice and chives in a small bowl and stir to mix well, then add to the salad and stir gently to coat.

Serve 1 pork cutlet per person with one-quarter of the mash and salad alongside.

12 G FIBRE PER SERVE **GOOD SOURCE OF RESISTANT STARCH**

UNITS PER SERVE ❋ BREADS AND CEREALS **1** ❋ PROTEIN **2** ❋ FRUIT **0** ❋ VEGETABLES **2** ❋ DAIRY **1** ❋ FATS AND OILS **2**

Beef and Lamb Mains

Balsamic-glazed steaks *with* roasted vegetable salad

SERVES 4
PREPARATION 15 minutes
COOKING 30 minutes, plus potato and sweet potato cooking time

----

olive oil spray, for cooking
2 × 400 g rump steaks, halved
    horizontally or 4 × 200 g minute
    steaks, all visible fat removed
2 tablespoons balsamic vinegar

ROASTED VEGETABLE SALAD
450 g chat potatoes, steamed,
    lightly crushed and chilled overnight
    (see page 41)
150 g sweet potato, cut into 2 cm
    pieces, steamed and chilled
    overnight (see page 41)
1 eggplant, cut into 3 cm pieces
1 large red capsicum, seeded and
    cut into 2 cm pieces
1½ tablespoons finely
    chopped rosemary
1 tablespoon garlic-infused olive oil
250 g grape or cherry tomatoes
1 large zucchini, halved lengthways and
    cut into 2 cm pieces

Preheat the oven to 210°C (190° fan-forced). Line a large roasting tin with baking paper.

To make the roasted vegetable salad, place the crushed potatoes, sweet potato, eggplant and capsicum in the lined tin, then sprinkle with 1 tablespoon of the rosemary and drizzle with the olive oil, tossing well to coat. Roast for 15 minutes, then add the tomatoes and zucchini and scatter with the remaining rosemary, tossing gently to coat. Roast for another 15 minutes or until the vegetables are tender and golden brown and the potatoes are crisp.

Meanwhile, pan-fry the steaks. Heat a large heavy-based frying pan over high heat, then spray with olive oil. Season both sides of the steaks well with freshly ground black pepper, then pan-fry for 2–3 minutes on each side for medium–rare or continue until cooked to your liking. Transfer to a plate, cover loosely with foil and set aside. Remove the pan from the heat, then add the balsamic vinegar and stir to scrape up any caught-on bits from the base of the pan. Add ¼ cup (60 ml) water and bring to a simmer over low heat, stirring to create a sauce. Return the steaks to the pan, remove from the heat, then turn to coat in the sauce.

Place a steak on each of 4 plates, then spoon any remaining balsamic mixture in the pan over the roasted vegetables and gently stir to mix. Divide the vegetables evenly among the plates and serve immediately.

----

11 G FIBRE PER SERVE   **LOW FODMAP**   **GOOD SOURCE OF RESISTANT STARCH**

UNITS PER SERVE ✸ BREADS AND CEREALS **1** ✸ PROTEIN **2** ✸ FRUIT **0** ✸ VEGETABLES **2** ✸ DAIRY **0** ✸ FATS AND OILS **0**

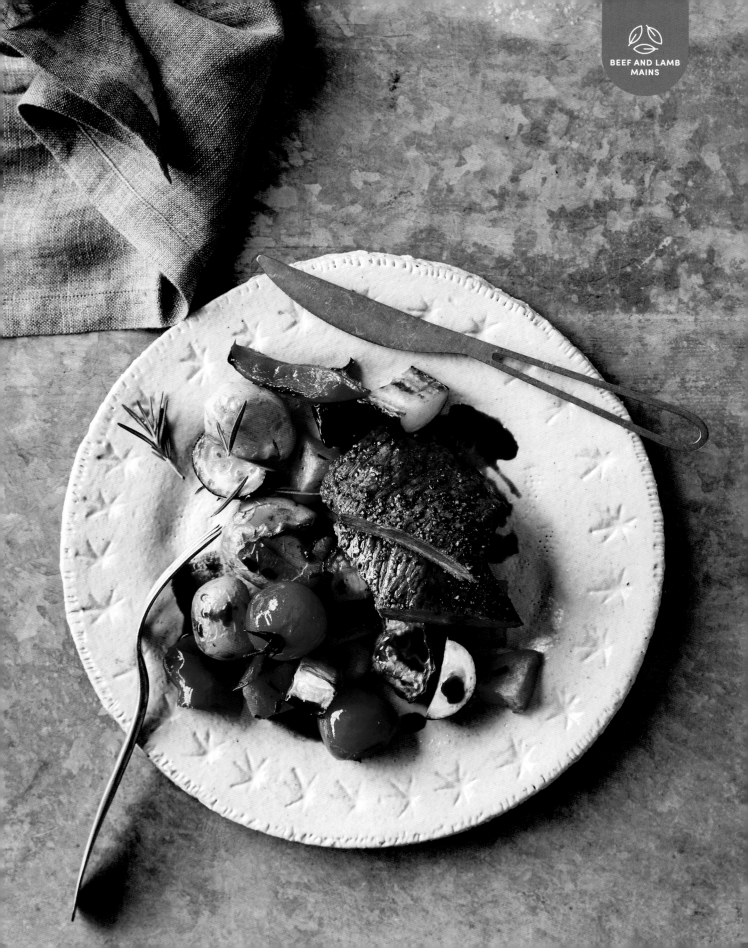

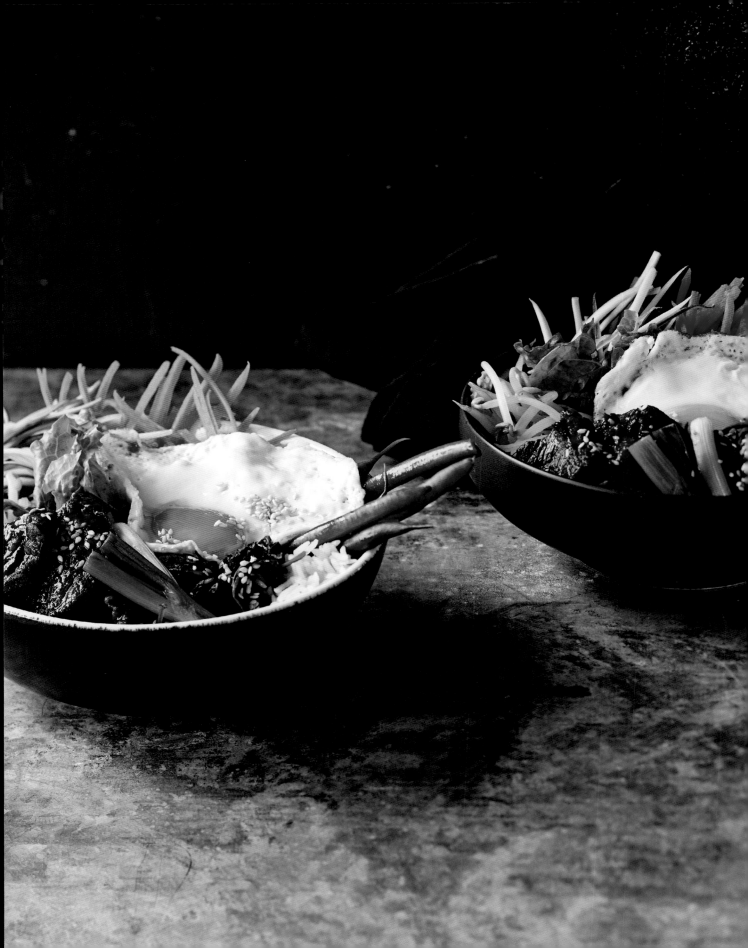

Bibimbap

SERVES 4
PREPARATION 25 minutes, plus 30 minutes marinating time
COOKING 25 minutes, plus rice cooking time

600 g rump steak, all visible
   fat removed, thinly sliced on
   the diagonal
1 tablespoon tamari (gluten-free
   soy sauce)
sesame oil, for drizzling
4 cups (300 g) baby spinach leaves,
   stems trimmed
1 tablespoon sesame seeds,
   lightly toasted
100 g bean sprouts, trimmed
2 carrots, cut into thin matchsticks
150 g green beans, trimmed
2 zucchini, cut into 5 cm long
   × 5 mm wide batons
olive oil spray, for cooking
2 spring onions (green tops only),
   cut into 4 cm lengths
4 eggs
1 cup (185 g) cooked basmati rice
   (see page 41)
1 baby cos lettuce, shredded

Place the beef in a bowl, add the tamari and drizzle with sesame oil, then stir to coat. Cover with plastic film and marinate in the refrigerator for at least 30 minutes.

Place the spinach in a small heavy-based saucepan with the water from washing still clinging to the leaves, then cover and place over high heat for 1 minute or until wilted. Remove and, when cool enough to handle, squeeze out as much liquid as possible. Place in a bowl and drizzle with sesame oil, then scatter with half of the sesame seeds. Set aside.

Working in batches, blanch the bean sprouts, carrot, green beans and zucchini in a saucepan of simmering water for 1–2 minutes until just tender. Set each vegetable aside in separate bowls.

Heat a wok over high heat and spray with olive oil. When the surface shimmers slightly, add one-third of the beef and cook on one side for 1 minute or until lightly browned, then turn the beef and cook on the other side for another minute or until browned. Transfer to a bowl. Spray the wok with oil and cook half of the remaining beef, then add to the bowl with the beef. Repeat with the remaining beef and the spring onion.

Heat a non-stick heavy-based frying pan over high heat. Spray with olive oil, then crack the eggs into the pan and cook for 3–4 minutes for sunny-side up or continue until cooked to your liking.

Divide the rice among 4 bowls, then, placing each ingredient in a small mound on top (the ingredients should be grouped), top with one-quarter of the beef mixture, spinach mixture, bean sprouts, carrot, green beans, zucchini and lettuce. Drizzle with sesame oil and scatter the beef with the remaining sesame seeds, then add an egg to each bowl and serve immediately.

9 G FIBRE PER SERVE   **LOW FODMAP**

UNITS PER SERVE ❋ BREADS AND CEREALS **1** ❋ PROTEIN **2** ❋ FRUIT **0** ❋ VEGETABLES **2** ❋ DAIRY **0** ❋ FATS AND OILS **1.5**

Chilli con carne *with* sweet potato *and* cannellini bean mash

SERVES 4
PREPARATION 20 minutes
COOKING 1 hour 40 minutes, plus sweet potato cooking time

olive oil spray, for cooking
800 g beef rump steak, all visible
    fat removed, cut into 2 cm cubes
2 sticks celery, finely chopped
1 carrot, finely chopped
1 tablespoon ground cumin
1 tablespoon sweet paprika
1½ teaspoons dried
    Greek-style oregano
1 × 400 g tin salt-reduced
    chopped tomatoes
4 salt-reduced chicken stock cubes
    dissolved in 3 cups (750 ml) boiling
    water, plus extra if needed
1 bay leaf
3 cups mixed salad leaves
250 g cherry tomatoes, halved
160 g avocado, sliced or diced

SWEET POTATO AND CANNELLINI BEAN MASH

200 g tinned cannellini beans,
    drained and rinsed
1 small sweet potato (about 400 g),
    roughly chopped, steamed and
    chilled overnight (see page 41)
1 teaspoon garlic-infused olive oil
1 tablespoon lactose-free
    natural yoghurt

Preheat the oven to 190°C (170°C fan-forced).

Heat an enamelled cast-iron casserole dish over medium heat and spray with olive oil. Working in 2 batches, cook the beef, stirring, for 4–5 minutes until browned all over, then transfer to a bowl. Add the celery and carrot to the dish and cook, stirring, for 3–4 minutes or until softened. Add the cumin, paprika and oregano and cook, stirring, for 30 seconds until fragrant, then return all the beef and any juices to the dish and stir to coat with the vegetable and spice mixture.

Add the tomatoes and stock and stir to combine, then bring to the boil. Add the bay leaf, then cover and transfer to the oven to cook for 1 hour 25 minutes or until the beef is tender; add a little extra stock or water to the dish if a thinner sauce is desired. Season to taste with freshly ground black pepper.

Meanwhile, to make the sweet potato and cannellini bean mash, place the cannellini beans in a heavy-based saucepan, cover with water and bring to the boil over high heat. Add the chilled sweet potato and olive oil, reduce the heat to low and simmer for 5 minutes to warm through. Drain well, then add the yoghurt and mash well with a vegetable masher (or use a stick blender to puree until smooth).

Divide the chilli con carne, mash, lettuce, tomatoes and avocado among 4 plates or shallow bowls and serve immediately.

13 G FIBRE PER SERVE   **GOOD SOURCE OF RESISTANT STARCH**

UNITS PER SERVE ❋ BREADS AND CEREALS **1** ❋ PROTEIN **2** ❋ FRUIT **0** ❋ VEGETABLES **2** ❋ DAIRY **1** ❋ FATS AND OILS **2**

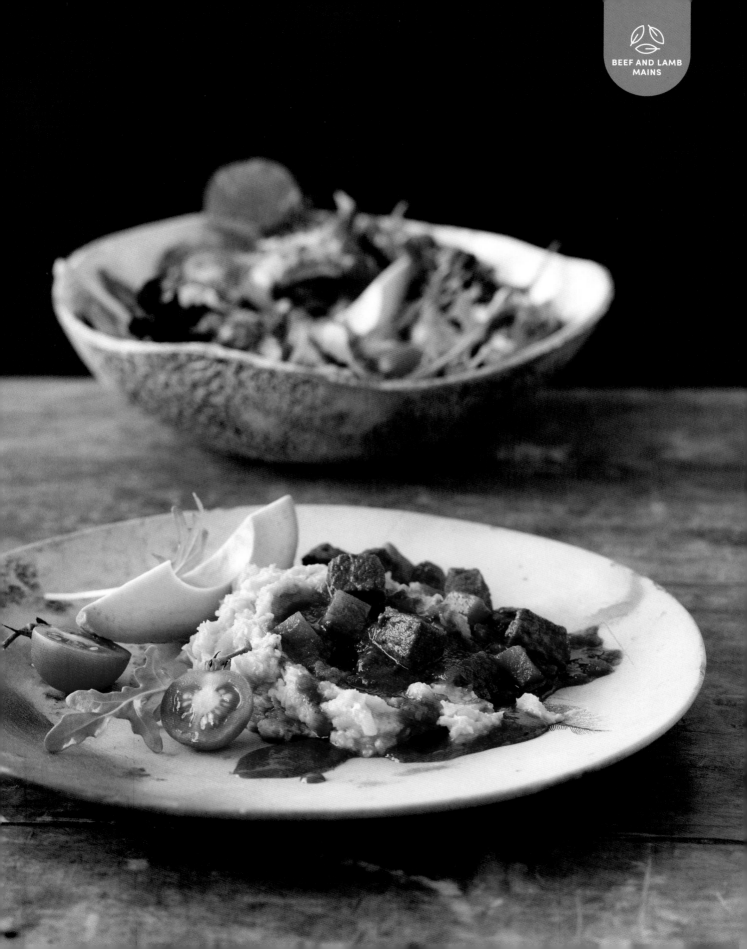

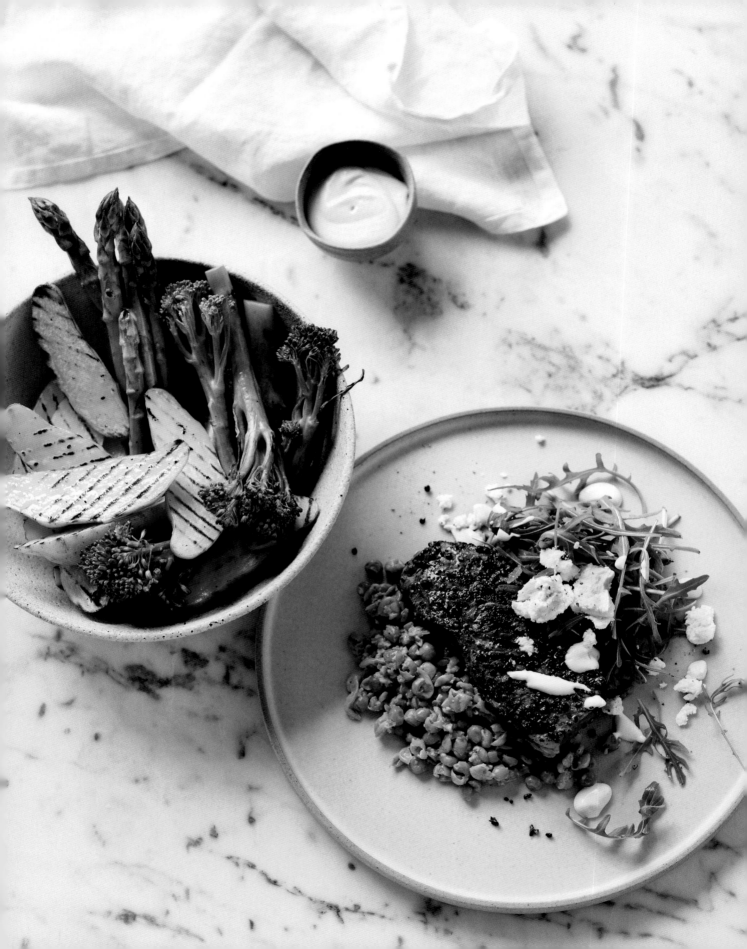

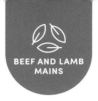
Pepper-crusted steaks *with* crushed peas *and* chargrilled vegetables

SERVES 4
PREPARATION 25 minutes
COOKING 35 minutes, plus potato cooking time

1½ tablespoons black peppercorns

1½ tablespoons dried
    green peppercorns

2 teaspoons whole allspice

4 × 200 g sirloin steaks, all visible
    fat removed

olive oil spray, for cooking

600 g kipfler potatoes, steamed,
    halved lengthways and chilled
    overnight (see page 41)

1 bunch asparagus, bases trimmed

1 bunch broccolini, bases trimmed,
    halved lengthways if large

⅓ cup (80 g) light sour cream

1 teaspoon Dijon mustard

150 g rocket leaves, trimmed

100 g goat's cheese, crumbled

CRUSHED PEAS

2 cups (240 g) frozen peas

1 tablespoon light sour cream

2 teaspoons finely grated lemon zest

Using a mortar and pestle, lightly crush the peppercorns and allspice, then place on a plate. Press both sides of the steaks on the pepper mixture to coat evenly. Set aside until ready to cook.

Heat a chargrill pan over medium–high heat, then spray with olive oil. Working in batches, chargrill the potato halves for 5–6 minutes on each side until warmed through and chargrill marks appear. Transfer to a plate and set aside. Sprinkle the asparagus with water, then add to the pan and chargrill for 1–2 minutes on each side until just tender and chargrill marks appear. Repeat with the broccolini.

Combine the sour cream and mustard in a small bowl. Cover with plastic film and refrigerate until required.

To make the crushed peas, cook the peas in a saucepan of simmering water for 3 minutes, then drain. Add the sour cream and crush lightly with a vegetable masher, then add the lemon zest and season to taste with freshly ground black pepper.

Spray the chargrill pan with olive oil. Cook the steaks for 3–4 minutes on each side for medium–rare or continue until cooked to your liking.

Divide the crushed peas among 4 plates and top each with a steak. Arrange one-quarter of the chargrilled vegetables, rocket and goat's cheese on each plate and either drizzle with the sour cream mixture or serve in a small bowl to the side. (Alternatively, place the grilled vegetables in a bowl, add the mustard sour cream and gently stir to combine, then scatter with the rocket and goat's cheese and divide among the plates.)

12 G FIBRE PER SERVE   **GOOD SOURCE OF RESISTANT STARCH**

UNITS PER SERVE ❋ BREADS AND CEREALS **1** ❋ PROTEIN **2** ❋ FRUIT **0** ❋ VEGETABLES **2** ❋ DAIRY **1** ❋ FATS AND OILS **1**

Coriander *and* lime-marinated steak *with* lentil, quinoa *and* watercress salad

SERVES 4
PREPARATION 25 minutes, plus 20 minutes marinating and 10 minutes cooling time
COOKING 30 minutes

¼ cup (60 g) lactose-free
    natural yoghurt
600 g rump steak, all visible fat
    removed, cut into 2 cm cubes
2 teaspoons tamari (gluten-free
    soy sauce)
olive oil spray, for cooking

CORIANDER AND LIME MARINADE
1 stick celery, chopped
2 spring onions (green tops only),
    roughly chopped
handful coriander leaves
1 fresh long red chilli, seeded and
    finely chopped
finely grated zest and juice of 1 lime

LENTIL, QUINOA AND WATERCRESS SALAD
½ cup (100 g) tri-colour quinoa,
    rinsed and drained
2 red capsicums, seeded and cut
    into quarters
200 g tinned salt-reduced lentils,
    drained and rinsed
150 g watercress sprigs
2 zucchini, sliced into rounds
200 g salt-reduced feta, crumbled
small handful coriander leaves,
    roughly chopped
1½ tablespoons lime juice
1 tablespoon extra virgin olive oil

To make the marinade, place all the ingredients in a blender and blend briefly until a coarse, chunky puree forms. Place ¼ cup (60 ml) of the puree in a small bowl, then stir in the yoghurt and mix until well combined. Cover with plastic film and refrigerate until required. Transfer the remaining marinade to a large bowl and add the beef. Add the tamari and stir to coat well. Cover with plastic film and marinate in the refrigerator for 20 minutes.

To make the salad, place the quinoa in a small heavy-based saucepan and cover with 1 cup (250 ml) water. Bring to the boil over medium heat, then reduce the heat to low, cover and cook for 10–12 minutes until most of the water has been absorbed and the quinoa is tender. Drain, if necessary, then transfer to a bowl and leave to cool for 10 minutes.

Meanwhile, preheat the oven grill to high. Place the capsicum, skin-side up, on a baking tray lined with foil, then grill for 8–10 minutes until softened and charred. Transfer to a bowl, cover with plastic film and leave to stand for 10 minutes, then peel off the skin and finely chop the flesh. Add the capsicum to the bowl of quinoa, then add the lentils, watercress, zucchini, feta, coriander, lime juice and olive oil and season to taste.

Just before serving, heat a heavy-based frying pan over high heat, then spray with olive oil. Working in batches, add the steak and sear for 2 minutes on each side for medium–rare or until cooked to your liking. Divide the steak evenly among 4 plates and serve with the quinoa salad and yoghurt sauce.

11 G FIBRE PER SERVE   **LOW FODMAP**   **GOOD SOURCE OF RESISTANT STARCH**

UNITS PER SERVE ❋ BREADS AND CEREALS **0.5** ❋ PROTEIN **2** ❋ FRUIT **0** ❋ VEGETABLES **2** ❋ DAIRY **1** ❋ FATS AND OILS **2**

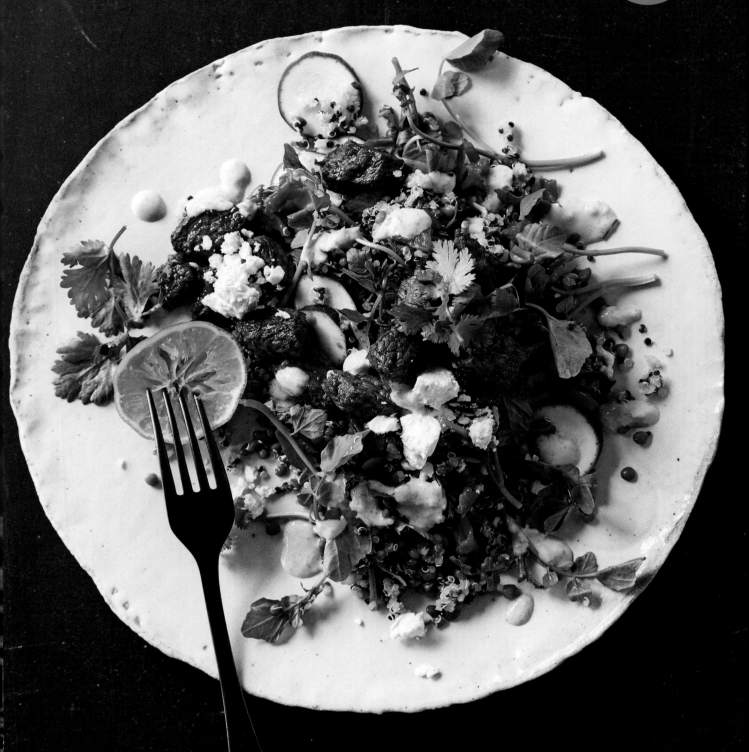

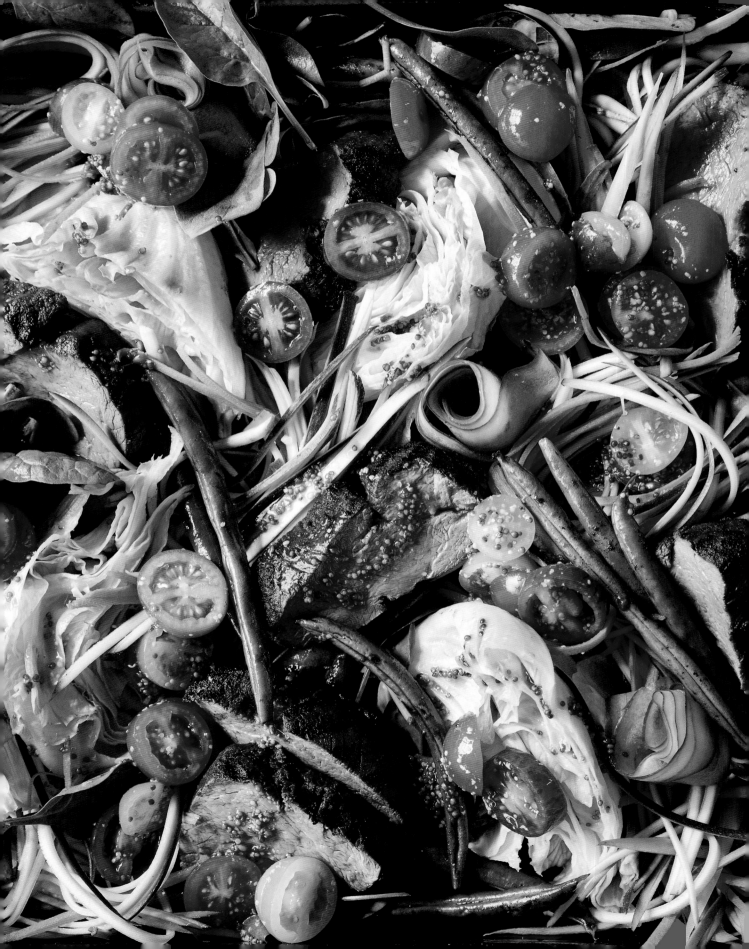

Smoky barbecued beef *and* vegetables *with* tomato dressing

SERVES 4
PREPARATION 20 minutes
COOKING 10 minutes, plus standing time

1 tablespoon garlic-infused olive oil
2 tablespoons red wine vinegar
1 tablespoon smoked or
    sweet paprika
4 x 200 g lean beef fillet steaks
100 g green beans , trimmed
1 carrot, cut into thin matchsticks
2 zucchini, cut into thin matchsticks
1 stick celery, cut into thin matchsticks
½ small iceberg lettuce, cut into wedges
1 cup baby spinach leaves
1 Lebanese cucumber, peeled into
    long thin ribbons

TOMATO DRESSING
125 g mixed cherry tomatoes, sliced
1 tablespoon garlic-infused olive oil
2 teaspoons wholegrain mustard
2 teaspoons pure maple syrup
2 tablespoons red wine vinegar

Preheat a barbecue chargrill plate and flat plate to high heat.

To make the tomato dressing, combine all the ingredients in a large bowl. Season to taste with freshly ground black pepper.

Place the olive oil, vinegar, paprika, steaks, green beans, carrot, zucchini and celery in a large bowl and toss until well coated. Using tongs, transfer the steaks to the barbecue chargrill plate and the vegetable mixture to the flat plate. Cook, turning the vegetables occasionally and the steaks only once, for 8–10 minutes for medium or until the beef is cooked to your liking. Divide the steaks and vegetables evenly among 4 serving plates, cover loosely with foil and rest for 3 minutes.

Add the iceberg lettuce, spinach and cucumber to the tomato dressing and toss gently to combine. Serve alongside the barbecued steak and vegetables.

7 G FIBRE PER SERVE   LOW FODMAP   GOOD SOURCE OF RESISTANT STARCH

UNITS PER SERVE ❋ BREADS AND CEREALS **0** ❋ PROTEIN **2** ❋ FRUIT **0** ❋ VEGETABLES **2.5** ❋ DAIRY **0** ❋ FATS AND OILS **2**

Cumin lamb *with* honeydew salad

SERVES 4
PREPARATION 20 minutes
COOKING 12 minutes, plus standing time

800 g lean lamb backstrap
1 tablespoon garlic-infused olive oil
3 teaspoons ground cumin
3 teaspoons ground coriander

HONEYDEW SALAD
1 tablespoon garlic-infused olive oil
finely grated zest and juice of 1 lemon
2 baby cos lettuces, leaves separated
1 cup small mint leaves
2 Lebanese cucumbers, thinly sliced
    into rounds
1 stick celery, thinly sliced
250 g cherry tomatoes, halved
200 g peeled, seeded and chopped
    honeydew melon
100 g salt-reduced Danish feta,
    crumbled

Preheat the oven grill to high and line a large baking tray with foil.

Place the lamb, olive oil, cumin and coriander in a large bowl and toss until well coated. Season to taste with freshly ground black pepper. Transfer to the prepared tray and cook under the grill, turning once, for 10–12 minutes for medium or until the lamb is cooked to your liking. Transfer to a chopping board, cover loosely with foil and rest for 3 minutes, then cut on the diagonal into thick slices.

Meanwhile, to make the honeydew salad, whisk together the olive oil, lemon zest and juice in a large bowl. Season to taste with freshly ground black pepper. Add the remaining ingredients and toss well to combine.

Divide the lamb evenly among 4 plates and serve with the honeydew salad.

You can serve this with 4 chargrilled slices of gluten-free chia and sunflower bread, drizzled with a little extra garlic-infused olive oil (this will add 1 unit of breads and cereals and 3 g fibre per serve).

8 G FIBRE PER SERVE   **LOW FODMAP**

UNITS PER SERVE ❋ BREADS AND CEREALS **0** ❋ PROTEIN **2** ❋ FRUIT **0.5** ❋ VEGETABLES **2.5** ❋ DAIRY **1** ❋ FATS AND OILS **2**

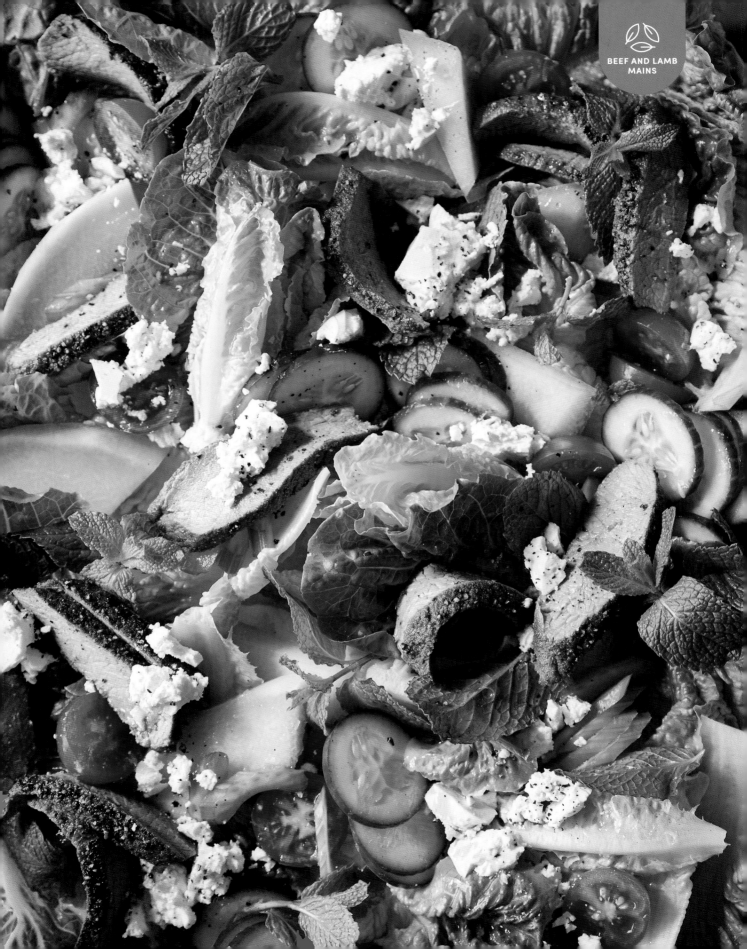

Lamb, spinach, potato *and* pea curry *with* spiced rice

SERVES 4
PREPARATION 20 minutes
COOKING 1 hour 15 minutes, plus potato cooking time

2 teaspoons garlic-infused olive oil
2 sticks celery, finely chopped
2 cm piece ginger, finely grated
2 teaspoons ground coriander
2 teaspoons ground cumin
½ teaspoon ground turmeric
¼ teaspoon ground cardamom
¼ teaspoon garam masala
pinch of ground cinnamon
800 g lean lamb leg steaks or fillet,
    all visible fat removed, cut into
    2 cm cubes
1 × 400 g tin salt-reduced
    chopped tomatoes
1 × 250 g packet frozen spinach, thawed
4 potatoes, cooked, chilled overnight,
    then cut into bite-sized pieces
    (see page 41)
120 g green beans, halved on
    the diagonal
lemon wedges, for squeezing

SPICED RICE
½ cup (100 g) brown basmati rice
1 teaspoon garlic-infused olive oil
1 small fresh red chilli, seeded
    and finely chopped
1 teaspoon finely grated ginger

Heat an enamelled cast-iron casserole or large heavy-based saucepan over medium heat and add the olive oil. Add the celery and cook, stirring for 3 minutes or until softened; add 1 tablespoon water to prevent the celery from sticking, if necessary. Add the ginger, coriander, cumin, turmeric, cardamom, garam masala and cinnamon and stir to combine, then cook for 30 seconds or until fragrant.

Add the lamb and cook, stirring, for 6–8 minutes until browned all over. Add the tomatoes and 2 cups (500 ml) water and bring to a simmer, then stir in the spinach. Reduce the heat to low and simmer, stirring occasionally, for 45 minutes. Add the potato and cook, covered, for 10 minutes to heat through. Add the green beans and cook, covered, for another 5 minutes or until the lamb is tender and the beans are cooked.

Meanwhile, to make the spiced rice, place the rice, 1½ cups (375 ml) water, the olive oil, chilli and ginger in a medium saucepan over high heat. Bring to the boil, then immediately reduce the heat to low. Cover and cook, gently simmering, for 15–20 minutes until the rice is tender and all the water is absorbed. Remove from the heat and leave to stand, covered, for 5 minutes. Fluff gently with a fork before serving.

Divide the spiced rice among 4 bowls and top each bowl with one-quarter of the curry. Serve with lemon wedges.

12 G FIBRE PER SERVE   LOW FODMAP   GOOD SOURCE OF RESISTANT STARCH

UNITS PER SERVE ❋ BREADS AND CEREALS **1** ❋ PROTEIN **2** ❋ FRUIT **0** ❋ VEGETABLES **2** ❋ DAIRY **0** ❋ FATS AND OILS **0.5**

Shepherd's pie *with* parsnip *and* cannellini mash

SERVES 4
PREPARATION 20 minutes
COOKING 1 hour 20 minutes, plus potato cooking time

olive oil spray, for cooking
1 onion, finely chopped
1 large carrot, finely chopped
1 stick celery, finely chopped
600 g lean minced lamb
2 tablespoons salt-reduced
    tomato paste
2 teaspoons Worcestershire sauce
1 teaspoon salt-reduced soy sauce
1½ tablespoons finely
    chopped rosemary
½ cup (125 ml) salt-reduced
    vegetable stock or water
1 bunch broccolini, trimmed
100 g green beans, trimmed

PARSNIP AND CANNELLINI MASH
1 parsnip, roughly chopped
600 g potatoes, quartered, steamed
    and chilled overnight (see page 41)
200 g tinned salt-reduced cannellini
    beans, drained and rinsed
2 tablespoons light sour cream
¼ cup (60 ml) skim milk, or as needed

Heat a heavy-based saucepan or enamelled cast-iron casserole dish over medium heat and spray with olive oil. Add the onion, carrot and celery and cook, stirring occasionally, for 4–5 minutes until softened. Add the lamb and, using a wooden spoon, stir to break up any clumps, then cook for 6–8 minutes until browned. Stir in the tomato paste, Worcestershire sauce, soy sauce and rosemary, then pour in the stock or water. Bring to the boil over high heat, then cover, reduce the heat to low and simmer for 25 minutes, stirring occasionally.

Meanwhile, to make the mash, cook the parsnip in a saucepan of simmering water over medium heat for 20 minutes or until tender, then drain well. Place in a bowl with the potato and cannellini beans and, using a vegetable masher, mash until smooth and well combined. Beat in the sour cream and enough milk as needed to form a smooth mash, then season to taste with freshly ground black pepper.

Preheat the oven to 200°C (180° fan-forced).

Transfer the lamb mixture to a 1.5 litre baking dish, then evenly spoon the mash over to cover. Run the tines of a fork over the mash to fluff it and create shallow ridges, then place on a baking tray. Bake for 40 minutes or until the top is golden and bubbling.

Steam the broccolini and beans in a steamer basket over a saucepan of simmering water for 5 minutes or until tender but still crisp.

Serve the shepherd's pie with the broccolini and beans alongside.

12 G FIBRE PER SERVE   **GOOD SOURCE OF RESISTANT STARCH**

UNITS PER SERVE   ❄ BREADS AND CEREALS **1**   ❄ PROTEIN **2**   ❄ FRUIT **0**   ❄ VEGETABLES **2**   ❄ DAIRY **0**   ❄ FATS AND OILS **1**

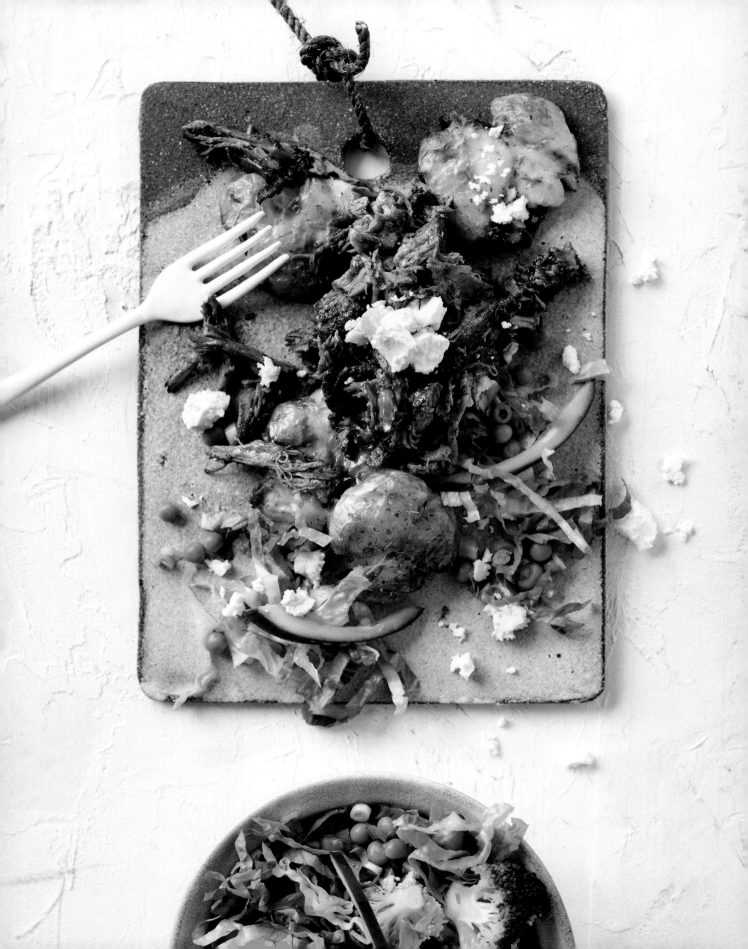

Slow-roasted lamb shawarma *with* crushed chat potatoes *and* salad

SERVES 4
PREPARATION 25 minutes
COOKING 2 hours 30 minutes, plus potato cooking time

2 teaspoons ground allspice
2 teaspoons sweet paprika
3 teaspoons dried Greek-style oregano
pinch of ground cinnamon
1 × 800 g boneless butterflied lamb leg, all visible fat trimmed
olive oil spray, for cooking
600 g chat potatoes, steamed, lightly crushed and chilled overnight (see page 41)
juice of 1 lemon
200 g salt-reduced low-fat feta, crumbled or diced

BROCCOLI, CUCUMBER AND PEA SALAD
½ small head broccoli, broken into florets
150 g frozen peas
1 baby cos lettuce, base trimmed, leaves washed, dried and shredded
1 Lebanese cucumber, halved lengthways, seeds removed, then thinly sliced on the diagonal
2 spring onions (green tops only), finely chopped
2 teaspoons lemon juice
1 teaspoon extra virgin olive oil

Preheat the oven to 190°C (170°C fan-forced).

Combine the allspice, paprika, 2 teaspoons of the oregano, the cinnamon and some freshly ground black pepper in a small bowl and rub all over the lamb to coat well. Place in a ceramic baking dish, then pour in enough water to come 2 cm up the side of the lamb, taking care not to pour it over the lamb. Spray the lamb with olive oil, then cover the dish tightly with foil. Roast for 2½ hours, checking the water occasionally and adding more if necessary. The lamb should be tender and easily shredded with a fork.

When the lamb has been cooking for 1½ hours, place the crushed potatoes in another roasting tin and pour the lemon juice evenly over the top. Spray with olive oil and sprinkle evenly with the remaining 1 teaspoon of oregano, then roast for 1 hour, turning occasionally, until golden and crisp.

Meanwhile, to make the salad, cook the broccoli in a saucepan of simmering water for 3 minutes, then add the peas and cook for another 2 minutes or until the vegetables are just tender. Drain and rinse under cold running water then set aside.

Just before serving, combine the broccoli, peas, cos, cucumber and spring onion in a bowl. Whisk together the lemon juice and olive oil, then add to the salad and toss to combine.

Shred the lamb with a fork, then serve 200 g per person with one-quarter each of the roast potatoes, salad and feta.

8 G FIBRE PER SERVE   **LOW FODMAP**   **GOOD SOURCE OF RESISTANT STARCH**

UNITS PER SERVE ❄ BREADS AND CEREALS **1** ❄ PROTEIN **2** ❄ FRUIT **0** ❄ VEGETABLES **2** ❄ DAIRY **1** ❄ FATS AND OILS **0**

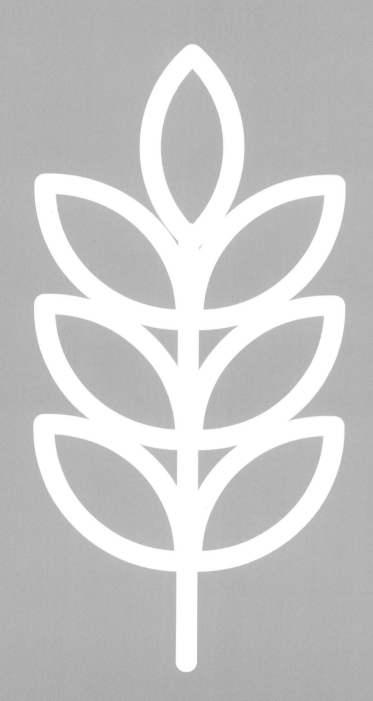

Vegetarian Mains

Lentil hotpot *with* steamed greens

SERVES 4
PREPARATION 20 minutes
COOKING 1 hour, plus potato cooking time

olive oil spray, for cooking
1 onion, finely chopped
1 large carrot, finely chopped
1 stick celery, finely chopped
1 large clove garlic, finely chopped
2 teaspoons curry powder
1 × 400 g tin salt-reduced
   chopped tomatoes
1 × 400 g tin lentils, drained and rinsed
1 × 400 g tin salt-reduced four-bean
   mix, drained and rinsed
1½ cups (180 g) frozen peas
5 potatoes, cut into 5 mm thick slices,
   steamed and chilled overnight
   (see page 41)
sweet paprika, for sprinkling
1 head broccoli, trimmed and cut
   into small florets
100 g green beans, trimmed

Preheat the oven to 190°C (170°C fan-forced). Spray a 1.5 litre baking dish with olive oil.

Heat a deep heavy-based frying pan over medium heat and spray with olive oil. Add the onion, carrot and celery and cook, stirring, for 5 minutes or until softened. Add the garlic and curry powder and stir for 30 seconds or until fragrant. Stir in the tomatoes, lentils and bean mix and bring to a simmer over medium–high heat, then stir in the peas and return to a simmer; add a little water if necessary to prevent the mixture from sticking.

Spoon the lentil mixture into the prepared baking dish, then top with the potato slices, placing them in overlapping lines to cover the lentil mixture. Spray with olive oil and sprinkle with paprika.

Bake the hotpot for 45–50 minutes until the potato topping is golden and crisp.

Just before serving, steam the broccoli and beans in a steamer basket over a saucepan of simmering water for 3 minutes or until tender but crisp. Serve the hotpot with the steamed vegetables alongside.

21 G FIBRE PER SERVE   **GOOD SOURCE OF RESISTANT STARCH**

UNITS PER SERVE ✻ BREADS AND CEREALS **1** ✻ PROTEIN **2** ✻ FRUIT **0** ✻ VEGETABLES **3** ✻ DAIRY **0** ✻ FATS AND OILS **0**

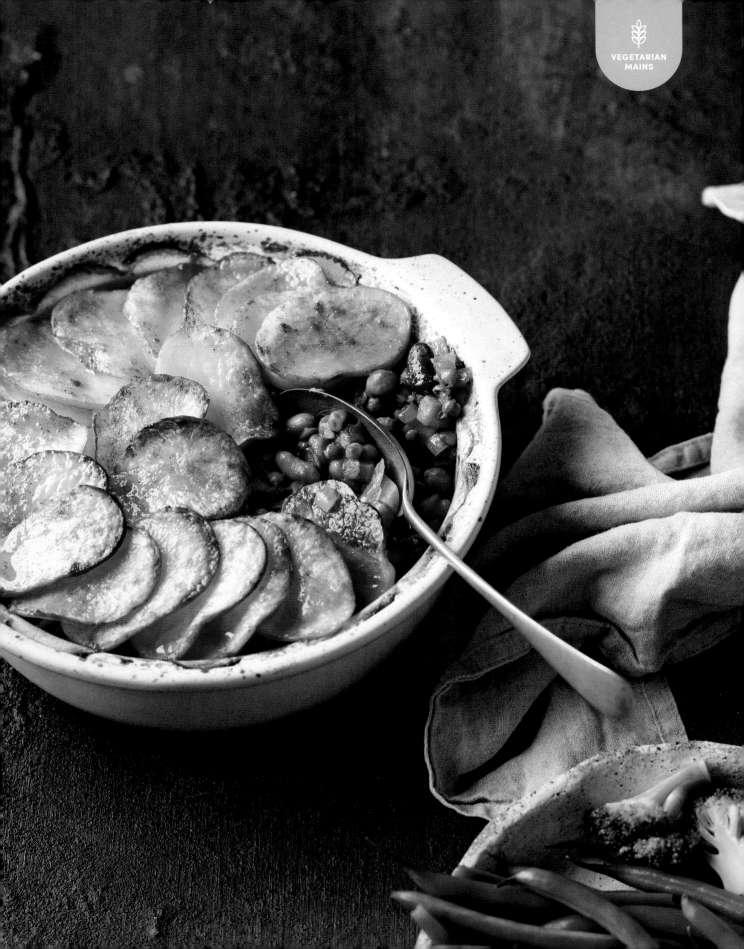

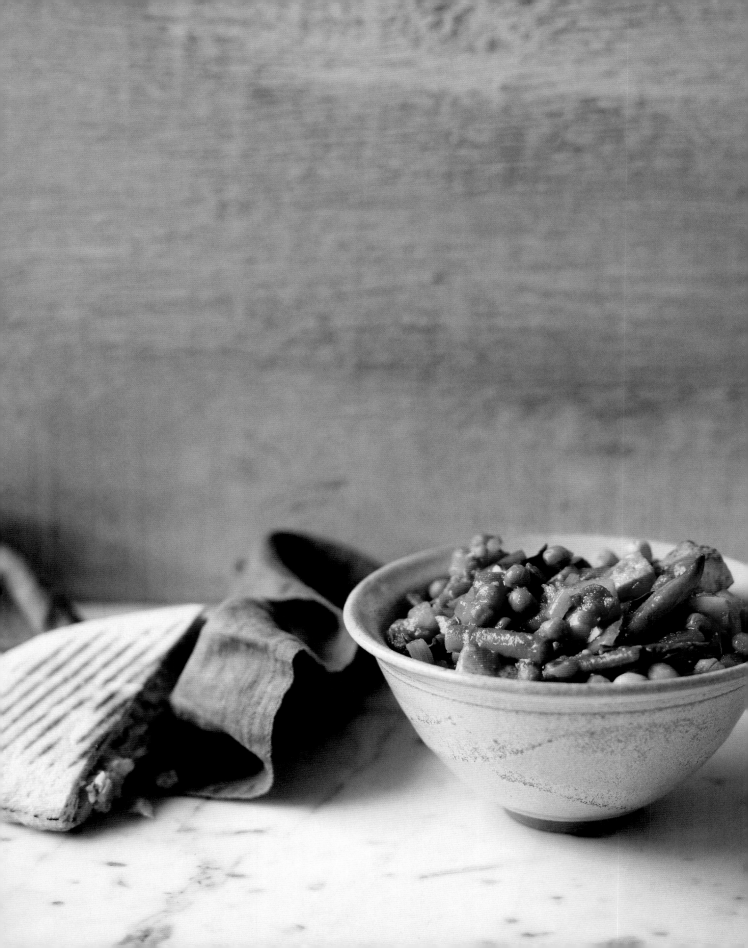

Potato *and* pea curry *with* chickpea *and* garlic flatbread

SERVES 4
PREPARATION 15 minutes
COOKING 40 minutes, plus potato cooking time

olive oil spray, for cooking
1 onion, finely chopped
1 clove garlic, finely chopped
1½ teaspoons finely grated ginger
2 teaspoons ground cumin
2 teaspoons ground coriander
1 teaspoon sweet paprika
½ teaspoon ground turmeric
1 × 400 g tin salt-reduced
    chopped tomatoes
100 g paneer, cut into 2 cm cubes
1 × 400 g tin salt-reduced chickpeas,
    drained and rinsed
1 potato, cut into 2 cm cubes, steamed
    and chilled overnight (see page 41)
2 cups (240 g) frozen peas
220 g green beans, trimmed and
    cut into 3 cm lengths
½ teaspoon garam masala
200 g baby spinach leaves, trimmed

CHICKPEA AND GARLIC FLATBREAD

1 × 400 g tin salt-reduced chickpeas,
    drained and rinsed
1 clove garlic, finely chopped
1 teaspoon lemon juice, or to taste
2 wholemeal pita bread pockets

Heat a large non-stick heavy-based frying pan over medium heat and spray with olive oil. Add the onion and cook for 5–6 minutes until softened and translucent. Add the garlic, ginger, cumin, coriander, paprika and turmeric and cook for another 30 seconds or until fragrant. Stir in the tomatoes and ½ cup (125 ml) water and cook for 15 minutes or until reduced and thickened.

Meanwhile, heat another non-stick heavy-based frying pan over medium heat and spray with olive oil. Working in batches so as not to crowd the pan, pan-fry the paneer for 2 minutes on each side or until golden. Drain on paper towel.

Add the chickpeas, paneer, potato, peas and beans to the curry, then partially cover and cook for 15 minutes or until the vegetables are tender, adding a little extra water to the pan, if needed, to prevent sticking.

Preheat the oven to 180°C (160°C fan-forced) and line a baking tray with baking paper.

To make the chickpea and garlic flatbread, place the chickpeas and garlic in a bowl and coarsely mash with a vegetable masher, then stir in lemon juice to taste. Divide the mashed chickpeas among the pita bread pockets, then place on the lined tray and bake for 4 minutes or until warmed through.

Stir the garam masala and spinach into the curry, then divide evenly among 4 bowls. Serve with half a pita bread pocket per person alongside.

19 G FIBRE PER SERVE   GOOD SOURCE OF RESISTANT STARCH

UNITS PER SERVE ❋ BREADS AND CEREALS **1** ❋ PROTEIN **2** ❋ FRUIT **0** ❋ VEGETABLES **2.5** ❋ DAIRY **1** ❋ FATS AND OILS **0**

Spiced black bean, corn *and* green rice bowl

SERVES 4
PREPARATION 25 minutes, plus overnight refrigerating and standing time
COOKING 35 minutes

1 small sweet potato (about 400 g)
1 teaspoon smoked sweet paprika
olive oil spray, for cooking
2 corn cobs, husks and silks removed
2 × 400 g tins reduced-salt black beans
    or kidney beans, drained and rinsed
2 teaspoons extra virgin olive oil
2 cloves garlic, finely chopped
⅓ cup (80 ml) lemon juice
½ teaspoon white balsamic vinegar
2 teaspoons ground cumin
80 g avocado, sliced
1 baby cos lettuce, trimmed and
    quartered lengthways
100 g mixed salad leaves
1 Lebanese cucumber, shaved
    lengthways into ribbons
100 g reduced-fat cheddar,
    coarsely grated
½ cup (125 g) light sour cream
coriander leaves and lime halves, to serve

GREEN RICE

1 cup (120 g) frozen peas
1 small onion, roughly chopped
1 fresh long green chilli, seeded
    and roughly chopped
2 cups (150 g) baby spinach leaves
⅓ cup mint leaves
⅓ cup flat-leaf parsley leaves
2 spring onions, roughly chopped
2 teaspoons olive oil
1 cup (185 g) cooked brown rice
    (see page 41)

Preheat the oven to 200°C (180°C fan-forced).

Cut the sweet potato into 1.5 cm dice, place in a bowl and add the paprika, then toss to coat well. Transfer to a roasting tin and spray with olive oil. Roast for 20 minutes, turning halfway, until golden and cooked through. Transfer to an airtight container and refrigerate overnight.

Place the corn in a saucepan, cover with cold water, then cover and bring to the boil. Remove from the heat and leave to stand for at least 15 minutes while you prepare the rice.

For the green rice, cook the peas in a saucepan of simmering water for 3 minutes or until tender. Drain and set aside. Process the onion, chilli, spinach, mint, parsley and spring onion in a food processor until a puree forms. Heat the olive oil in a heavy-based saucepan over medium heat, then add the green puree and cook, stirring, for 2–3 minutes until fragrant. Add the cooked rice and stir to coat in the puree, then add the peas and gently stir into the green rice.

Just before serving, place the drained beans in a small heavy-based saucepan, cover with water and bring to the boil, then boil for 1 minute. Drain and return to the cleaned pan, then add the olive oil, garlic, lemon juice, vinegar and cumin and heat over medium heat to warm the dressing through. Drain the corn, then carefully slice the kernels off the cobs in sections and add to the bean mixture.

Divide the rice among 4 bowls, then top with one-quarter of the bean and corn mixture, sweet potato, avocado, cos, salad leaves, cucumber, cheese and sour cream. Scatter with coriander, if using, and serve.

23 G FIBRE PER SERVE   **GOOD SOURCE OF RESISTANT STARCH**

UNITS PER SERVE ❋ BREADS AND CEREALS **1** ❋ PROTEIN **2** ❋ FRUIT **0** ❋ VEGETABLES **2** ❋ DAIRY **1** ❋ FATS AND OILS **3**

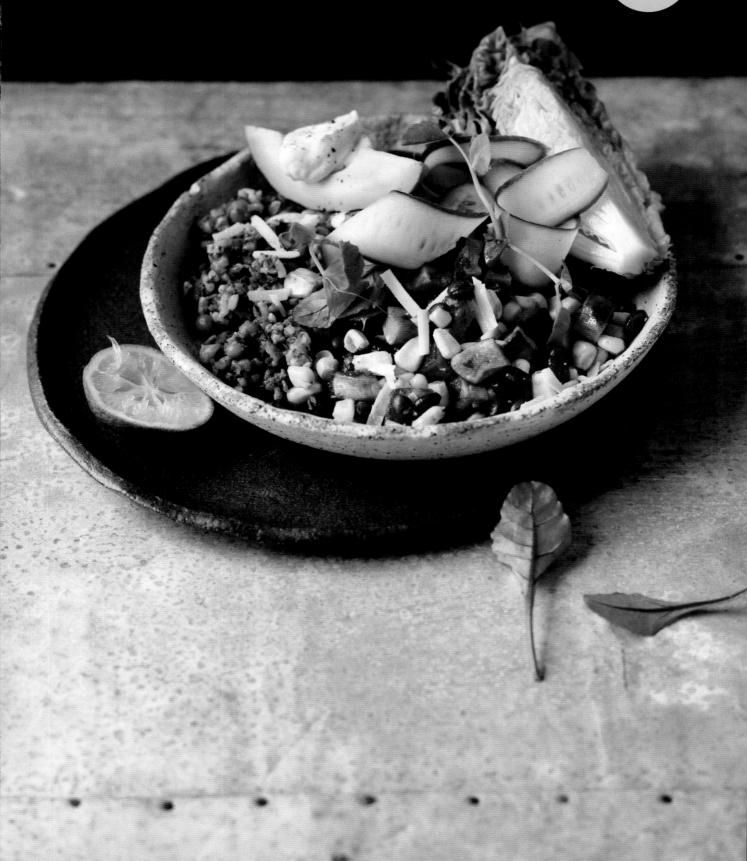

Spaghetti *with* lentil *and* mushroom 'meatballs', *and* cannellini bean *and* radicchio salad

SERVES 4
PREPARATION 20 minutes, plus cooling time
COOKING 50 minutes

½ cup (100 g) brown lentils
225 g button mushrooms,
    roughly chopped
2 cloves garlic, finely chopped
olive oil spray, for cooking
½ cup (125 ml) salt-reduced
    vegetable stock
½ teaspoon dried Greek-style oregano
40 g raw natural rolled oats
1 tablespoon LSA
1 tablespoon plain flour
2 tablespoons roughly chopped
    flat-leaf parsley leaves
1 small onion, finely chopped
1 carrot, coarsely grated
1 teaspoon sweet paprika
1 cup (250 ml) salt-reduced
    tomato passata
80 g spaghetti
finely grated parmesan, to serve

CANNELLINI BEAN AND RADICCHIO SALAD
2 cups mixed salad leaves
1 small head radicchio, leaves
    separated and torn
600 g tinned salt-reduced cannellini
    beans, drained and rinsed
3 teaspoons extra virgin olive oil
2 teaspoons lemon juice

Place the lentils in a heavy-based saucepan, cover with water and bring to the boil over high heat, then simmer over medium heat for 10 minutes. Drain, then place them, along with the mushrooms and half the garlic, in a food processor and pulse until finely chopped.

Preheat the oven to 180°C (160°C fan-forced). Line a 12-hole muffin tin with paper cases and spray well with olive oil.

Heat a non-stick heavy-based frying pan over medium heat and spray with olive oil. Add the lentil mixture, stock, oregano and oats and cook over medium heat, stirring constantly, for 5 minutes or until all the liquid is absorbed. Leave to cool slightly then mix in the LSA, flour and parsley. Divide into 12 portions then roll into balls. Place a ball in each lined muffin hole, then bake for 40 minutes or until golden.

Meanwhile, heat a heavy-based frying pan with a lid over medium heat and spray with olive oil. Add the onion and carrot and cook for 5 minutes. Add the sweet paprika and remaining garlic and cook for 30 seconds or until fragrant. Pour in the passata and ¼ cup (60 ml) water and bring to the boil. Reduce the heat to low, then cover and simmer for 20 minutes.

To make the salad, place the salad leaves, radicchio and beans in a bowl and toss gently to combine. Just before serving, add the olive oil and lemon juice and toss again.

Bring a large saucepan of water to the boil, cook the spaghetti according to the packet instructions, then drain. Stir the drained spaghetti and 'meatballs' through the tomato sauce to coat. Serve with the salad alongside, and finish with grated parmesan.

19 G FIBRE PER SERVE   **GOOD SOURCE OF RESISTANT STARCH**

UNITS PER SERVE   ❋ BREADS AND CEREALS **1**   ❋ PROTEIN **2**   ❋ FRUIT **0**   ❋ VEGETABLES **3**   ❋ DAIRY **0**   ❋ FATS AND OILS **0**

Braised Indian-style potato, zucchini, eggplant *and* lentils

SERVES 4
PREPARATION 15 minutes
COOKING 30 minutes, plus potato cooking time

olive oil spray, for cooking
2 sticks celery, finely chopped
2 teaspoons finely grated ginger
1½ teaspoons mustard seeds
1 teaspoon ground cumin
1 teaspoon ground coriander
1 teaspoon ground turmeric
pinch of chilli powder (optional)
1 sprig curry leaves (optional)
2 potatoes (about 250 g), cut into
   1.5 cm dice, steamed and chilled
   overnight (see page 41)
4 zucchini, cut into 3 cm pieces
1 eggplant, cut into 3 cm pieces
150 g green beans, trimmed and
   halved on the diagonal
1 × 400 g tin salt-reduced lentils,
   drained and rinsed
2 cups (150 g) baby spinach
   leaves, trimmed
4 eggs
coriander leaves, to serve (optional)

Heat a deep non-stick heavy-based frying pan over medium heat and spray with olive oil. Add the celery and cook for 3 minutes or until softened. Stir in the ginger, mustard seeds, cumin, coriander, turmeric and chilli powder and curry leaves, if using, and cook for 30 seconds or until fragrant.

Add the potato, zucchini and eggplant and cook for 2–3 minutes, stirring to coat in the spiced onion mixture. Add ½ cup (125 ml) hot water and bring to the boil, then reduce the heat to low, cover and simmer for 10–15 minutes until the vegetables are tender. Stir in the green beans, lentils and spinach, add a little extra water if necessary to prevent the vegetables from sticking, then return to a simmer and cook for another 3 minutes or until the beans are tender and the lentils are warmed through; the sauce should be thick.

Meanwhile, heat a non-stick heavy-based frying pan over medium heat and spray with olive oil. Break in the eggs and fry for 3 minutes for sunny-side up, or turn and cook for another 2 minutes or until cooked to your liking.

Divide the braised potato mixture and eggs among 4 plates or bowls. Scatter with coriander, if using, and serve.

14 G FIBRE PER SERVE   LOW FODMAP   GOOD SOURCE OF RESISTANT STARCH

UNITS PER SERVE   BREADS AND CEREALS **1**   PROTEIN **2**   FRUIT **0**   VEGETABLES **2**   DAIRY **0**   FATS AND OILS **1**

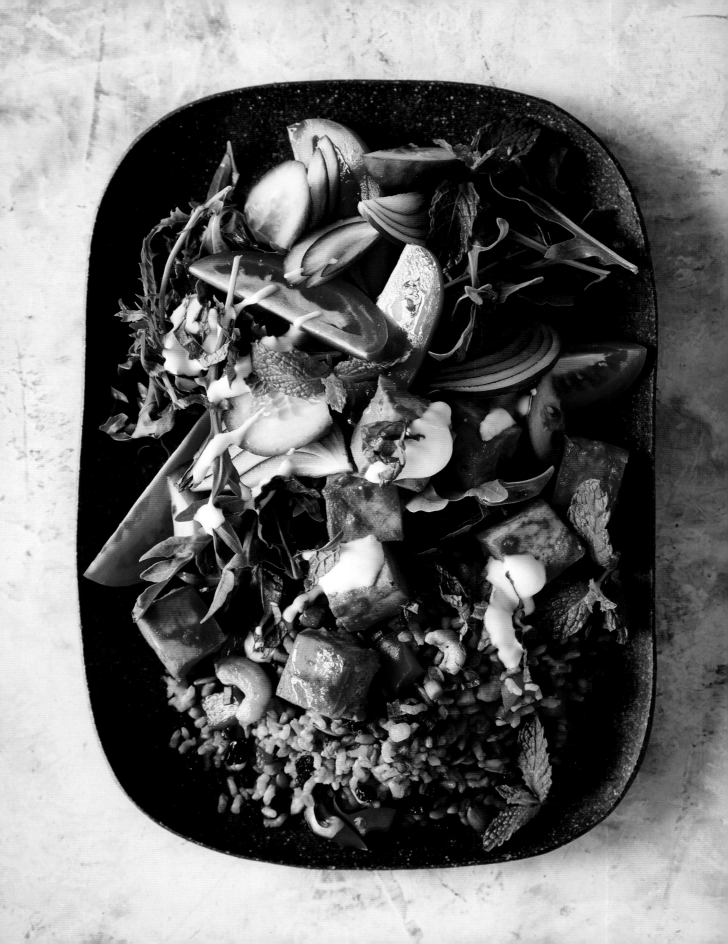

Tandoori tofu *with* tomato, cucumber *and* mint salad

SERVES 4
PREPARATION TIME 20 minutes, plus 15 minutes pressing and 15 minutes marinating time
COOKING TIME 20 minutes

800 g firm tofu, drained
olive oil spray, for cooking
1 quantity Brown Rice, Capsicum,
    Currant and Cashew Salad
    (see page 89)

TANDOORI MARINADE

⅓ cup (80 g) reduced-fat
    natural Greek-style yoghurt
1 small onion, finely chopped
2 cloves garlic, crushed
1 × 50 g sachet salt-reduced
    tomato paste
3 teaspoons ground cumin
3 teaspoons ground coriander
3 teaspoons sweet paprika
½ teaspoon ground ginger
½ teaspoon ground turmeric
¼ teaspoon smoked paprika
¼ teaspoon ground cardamom

TOMATO, CUCUMBER AND MINT SALAD

4 roma tomatoes, cut into thin wedges
2 Lebanese cucumbers, cut into
    chunks on the diagonal
½ small red onion, cut into thin wedges
120 g rocket leaves, trimmed
⅓ cup (80 g) reduced-fat natural
    Greek-style yoghurt
2 tablespoons thinly sliced mint leaves

Press the tofu between 2 plates or heavy-based baking trays for 15 minutes.

Meanwhile, to make the marinade, place all the ingredients in a food processor or blender and blend to combine.

Cut the pressed tofu into 2 cm cubes and place in a baking dish, then spoon the marinade over, turning to coat evenly. Season with freshly ground black pepper and set aside for 15 minutes to marinate.

Preheat the oven to 210°C (190°C fan-forced).

Line a baking tray with baking paper, then place an ovenproof wire rack on top. Place the tofu on the wire rack and spray with olive oil, then bake for 7 minutes or until golden brown. Turn, spray again with oil and bake for another 7 minutes or until slightly charred. Preheat the oven grill to high and grill for 2 minutes on each side or until well browned.

While the tofu is cooking, make the salad. Place the tomato, cucumber, onion and rocket in a bowl and stir gently to mix. Place the yoghurt and mint in a small bowl and stir to combine. Just before serving, add the yoghurt dressing to the salad and gently mix to lightly coat.

Divide the rice salad and tomato salad among 4 plates and top each with one-quarter of the tofu, then serve.

20 G FIBRE PER SERVE   **GOOD SOURCE OF RESISTANT STARCH**

UNITS PER SERVE   BREADS AND CEREALS **1**   PROTEIN **2**   FRUIT **0**   VEGETABLES **3**   DAIRY **0.5**   FATS AND OILS **0.5**

Asian barley pilaf *with* steamed greens

SERVES 4
PREPARATION 15 minutes
COOKING 45 minutes

3 cups (750 ml) salt-reduced
    vegetable stock
1 star anise
olive oil spray, for cooking
1 red onion, finely chopped
1 large clove garlic, finely chopped
1.5 cm piece ginger, finely grated
¼ teaspoon five-spice powder,
    or to taste
1½ cups (300 g) pearl barley,
    rinsed and drained
1 cup (120 g) frozen peas
1 bunch choy sum, trimmed and cut
    into 4 cm lengths
1 bunch broccolini, trimmed and cut
    into 4 cm lengths
150 g sugar snap peas, trimmed
150 g green beans, trimmed and
    halved on the diagonal
3 teaspoons salt-reduced soy sauce
    or tamari (gluten-free soy sauce)
sesame oil, for drizzling
100 g fresh shiitake mushrooms,
    trimmed and sliced
4 eggs, lightly beaten
600 g firm tofu, cut into 1.5 cm thick
    slices, patted dry with paper towel

Place the stock and star anise in a heavy-based saucepan and bring to a simmer. Cover and keep at a very low simmer.

Heat another heavy-based saucepan over medium heat and spray with olive oil. Add the onion and cook, stirring, for 5 minutes or until softened and translucent, then add the garlic, ginger and five-spice and cook for 30 seconds or until fragrant. Strain the hot stock, discarding the star anise, and add to the pan, along with the barley. Bring to a simmer, then reduce the heat to low and cook, covered, for 30–35 minutes until all the liquid is absorbed and the barley is tender but still a little chewy.

Meanwhile, cook the peas in a saucepan of simmering water for 3 minutes or until tender. Drain and set aside.

Working in batches, steam the choy sum, broccolini, sugar snaps and beans in a steamer basket over a saucepan of simmering water for 3–4 minutes until just tender. Add the peas to the steamed greens, then drizzle with the soy sauce and sesame oil.

Heat a non-stick heavy-based frying pan over medium heat and spray with olive oil. Add the mushrooms and cook, stirring for 2–3 minutes until tender and golden. Add to the greens. Spray the pan with olive oil, add the egg and cook for 1–2 minutes until the bottom has set, then carefully flip over and cook for another 1 minute or until golden and dry. Transfer the omelette to a chopping board, roll up and cut into 1 cm thick slices.

Heat the frying pan over medium heat and spray with olive oil. Cook the tofu for 3 minutes on each side or until golden.

Divide the pilaf and vegetables evenly among 4 bowls, then top with one-quarter of the omelette and tofu and serve immediately.

21 G FIBRE PER SERVE **GOOD SOURCE OF RESISTANT STARCH**

UNITS PER SERVE ✸ BREADS AND CEREALS **1** ✸ PROTEIN **2** ✸ FRUIT **0** ✸ VEGETABLES **2** ✸ DAIRY **0** ✸ FATS AND OILS **0**

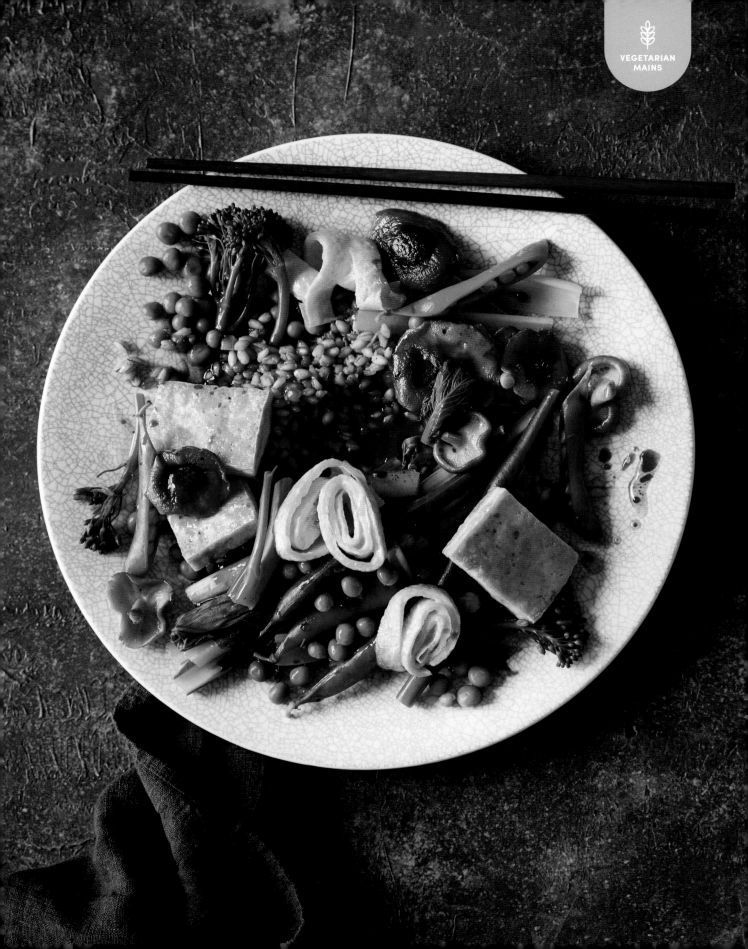

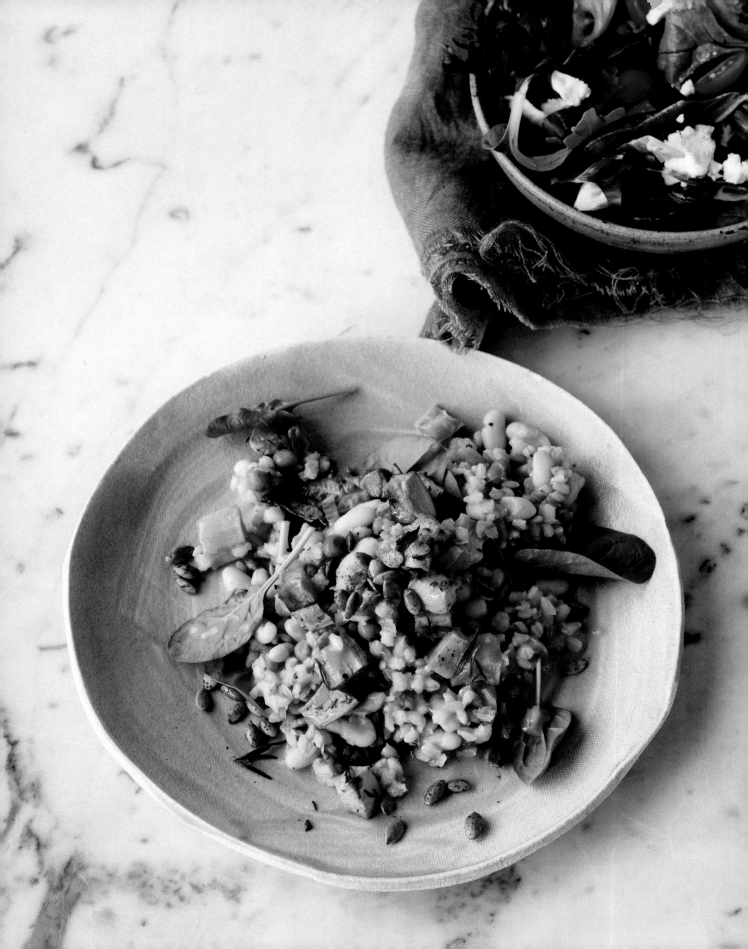

VEGETARIAN
MAINS

Barley risotto *with* roasted pumpkin, sweet potato, spinach *and* feta

SERVES 4
PREPARATION 20 minutes, plus refrigerating and standing time
COOKING 1 hour 5 minutes

1 small sweet potato (about 400 g),
　cut into 1.5 cm dice
200 g seeded, peeled butternut or Kent
　pumpkin, cut into 1.5 cm dice
olive oil spray, for cooking
2 teaspoons finely chopped rosemary
3 cups (750 ml) salt-reduced
　vegetable stock
1 leek, white part only, finely chopped
1 clove garlic, finely chopped
1½ cups (300 g) pearl barley,
　rinsed and drained
2 × 400 g tins salt-reduced cannellini
　beans, drained and rinsed
¼ cup (35 g) pumpkin seeds (pepitas)
¼ teaspoon sweet paprika
1 cup (120 g) frozen peas
100 g baby spinach leaves, trimmed
　and shredded
200 g mixed salad leaves
1 small radicchio, leaves torn
250 g grape tomatoes, halved
extra virgin olive oil, for drizzling
squeeze of lemon juice
160 g salt-reduced feta, crumbled
　or diced

Preheat the oven to 200°C (180° fan-forced). Line a baking tray with baking paper, add the sweet potato and pumpkin pieces, spray with olive oil and scatter with the rosemary. Roast for 20–25 minutes until tender. Once cool, refrigerate overnight in an airtight container.

Place the stock in a heavy-based saucepan and bring to a simmer. Cover and keep at a very low simmer.

Heat another heavy-based saucepan over medium heat and spray with olive oil. Add the leek and cook, stirring, for 5 minutes or until softened, then add the garlic and cook for 30 seconds. Stir in the barley and hot stock and bring to a simmer. Reduce the heat to low, then cover and cook for 30 minutes until most of the liquid is absorbed and the barley is tender but still slightly chewy. Stir in the cannellini beans, then cook for 2–3 minutes. Remove from the heat, cover and leave to stand for 5 minutes.

Meanwhile, preheat the oven to 180°C (160°C fan-forced). Place the pumpkin seeds on a baking tray, sprinkle with the paprika and spray with olive oil. Roast for 5 minutes or until golden and toasted, then set aside to cool. Transfer the chilled sweet potato and pumpkin to a baking tray lined with baking paper and place in the oven for 6 minutes or until warmed through.

Cook the peas in a saucepan of simmering water for 3 minutes, then drain. Add the roasted vegetables, peas and spinach to the risotto and gently stir to combine. Cover and leave to stand for 5 minutes. Place the salad leaves, radicchio and tomatoes in a bowl, drizzle with a little olive oil and a squeeze of lemon juice. Divide the risotto among 4 bowls and scatter the pumpkin seeds and feta over the top. Serve immediately with the salad alongside.

25 G FIBRE PER SERVE　**GOOD SOURCE OF RESISTANT STARCH**

UNITS PER SERVE ❋ BREADS AND CEREALS **1** ❋ PROTEIN **2** ❋ FRUIT **0** ❋ VEGETABLES **3** ❋ DAIRY **1** ❋ FATS AND OILS **2**

Peppered tofu *and* eggplant stir-fry

SERVES 4
PREPARATION 20 minutes
COOKING 5 minutes

2 tablespoons macadamia oil
800 g firm tofu, sliced
1 eggplant, chopped
3 teaspoons freshly ground
    black pepper
5 cm piece ginger, cut into
    thin matchsticks
½ bunch choy sum, cut into
    5 cm lengths
1 tablespoon tamari (gluten-free
    soy sauce)
1 carrot, cut into thin matchsticks
1 stick celery, cut into thin matchsticks

Heat the macadamia oil in a large wok over high heat. Add the tofu, eggplant, pepper and ginger and stir-fry for 2–3 minutes until the eggplant is soft and everything looks caramelised.

Add the choy sum and 1 tablespoon water and stir-fry for 30 seconds until it is just starting to wilt. Immediately remove the wok from the heat and toss through the tamari, carrot and celery. Leave to stand for 1 minute, then toss well and serve.

If desired, you can serve this stir-fry with raw zucchini noodles, made from 2 zucchini.

11 G FIBRE PER SERVE   **LOW FODMAP**

UNITS PER SERVE ✳ BREADS AND CEREALS **0** ✳ PROTEIN **2** ✳ FRUIT **0** ✳ VEGETABLES **1.5** ✳ DAIRY **0** ✳ FATS AND OILS **2**

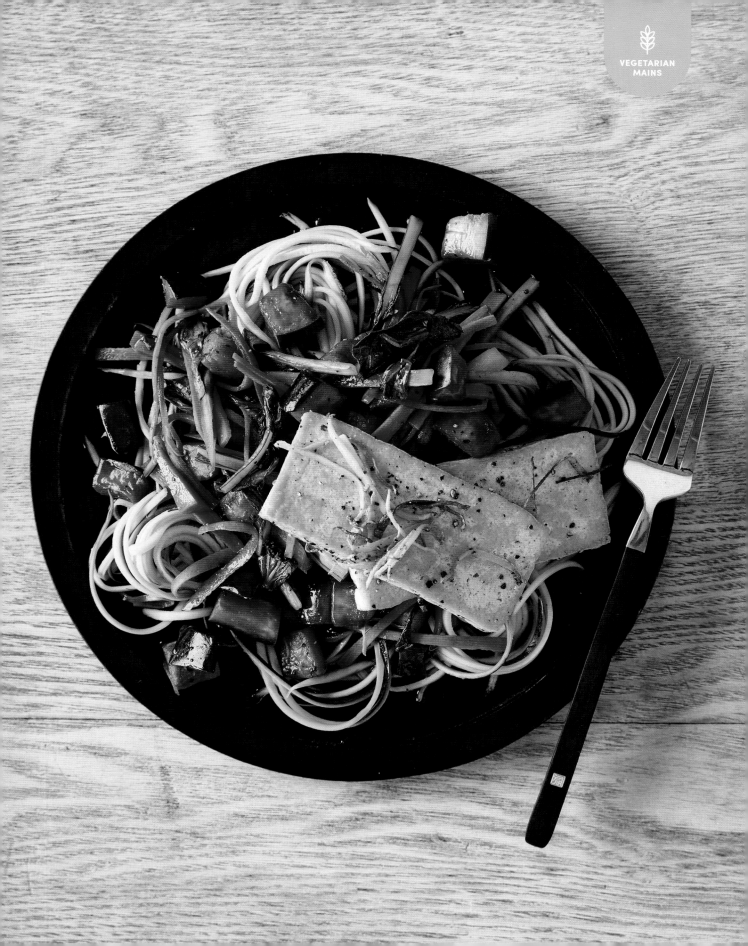

Snacks

Banana and oat pikelets with yoghurt

SERVES 6
PREPARATION 15 minutes, plus soaking time
COOKING 15 minutes

You can use the same amount of potato starch in place of the green banana flour if you like.

⅓ cup (50 g) raw (natural) rolled oats
up to ¾ cup (100 g) green banana flour
1 teaspoon baking powder
¼ teaspoon freshly grated nutmeg
1 cup (250 ml) high-calcium,
    lactose-free skim milk
1 egg, lightly beaten
2 bananas, mashed
olive oil spray, for cooking
2 large bananas, extra, sliced
600 g lactose-free natural yoghurt

Place the oats in a food processor and process until finely chopped to a flour texture. Transfer to a measuring jug and add enough green banana flour to make 1 cup total (100 g) flour.

Place the flour mixture in a large bowl, add the baking powder and nutmeg and whisk to combine. Whisk in the milk and egg to form a batter, then fold in the mashed banana.

Heat a large non-stick heavy-based frying pan over low–medium heat and spray with olive oil. Working in batches so as not to crowd the pan, add 1 tablespoon of batter for each pikelet and cook for 1–2 minutes until bubbles start to appear on the surface. Carefully turn over and cook for another 1–2 minutes until golden. Transfer to a heatproof plate and repeat with the remaining batter, spraying with a little more oil if needed. You should have enough batter to make 24 pikelets.

Serve the pikelets with the sliced banana and yoghurt alongside. (Any leftover pikelets can be stored in a single layer in an airtight container in the refrigerator for 1 day.)

6 G FIBRE PER SERVE   **LOW FODMAP**   **GOOD SOURCE OF RESISTANT STARCH**

UNITS PER SERVE ❁ BREADS AND CEREALS **2** ❁ PROTEIN **0** ❁ FRUIT **1** ❁ VEGETABLES **0** ❁ DAIRY **1** ❁ FATS AND OILS **0**

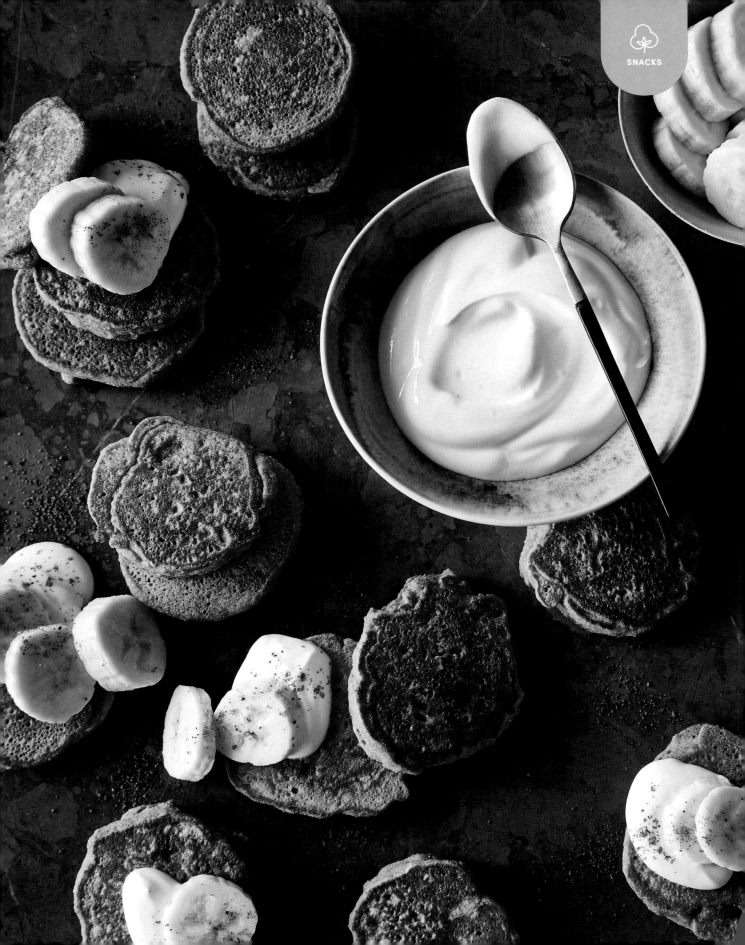

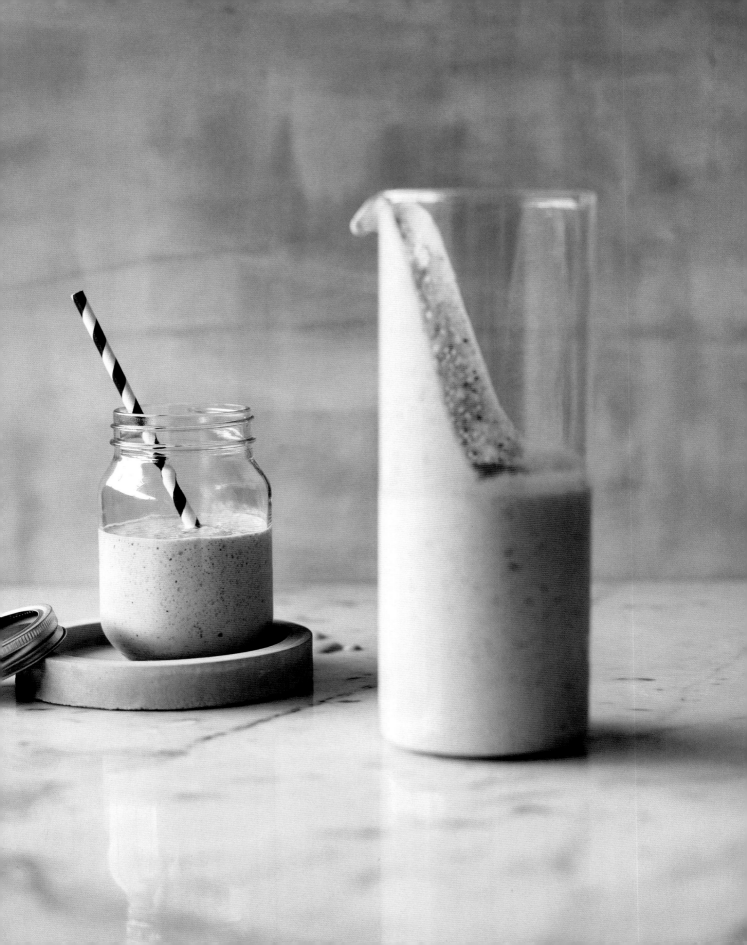

Banana, berry *and* yoghurt smoothie

SERVES 4
PREPARATION 5 minutes
COOKING Nil

1 banana
2 cups (400 g) frozen mixed berries
600 g lactose-free natural yoghurt
1½ cups (375 ml) high-calcium,
   lactose-free skim milk
1½ tablespoons green banana flour

Place all the ingredients in a blender and blend until smooth.
Pour evenly into 4 glasses and serve.

6 G FIBRE PER SERVE **LOW FODMAP** **GOOD SOURCE OF RESISTANT STARCH**

UNITS PER SERVE ✱ BREADS AND CEREALS **0** ✱ PROTEIN **0** ✱ FRUIT **1** ✱ VEGETABLES **0** ✱ DAIRY **1** ✱ FATS AND OILS **0**

Cinnamon granola bars

MAKES 12
PREPARATION 10 minutes
COOKING 25 minutes

½ cup (70 g) reduced-sugar
    dried cranberries
1½ cups (185 g) Cinnamon, Cashew
    and Dried Cranberry Granola
    (see page 64)

Preheat the oven to 160°C (140°C fan-forced). Line an 18 cm square cake tin with baking paper, leaving enough overhanging on 2 sides to lift out the baked slice.

Place the dried cranberries in a blender, add ½ cup (125 ml) water and blend until a smooth puree forms.

Place the granola in a bowl, add the cranberry puree and fold to combine well. Transfer the mixture to the lined tin, smoothing the surface with a flexible spatula.

Bake for 20–25 minutes until golden and firm. Leave to cool completely in the tin, then lift out onto a chopping board and cut into 12 bars. Store in an airtight container for up to 5 days.

3 G FIBRE PER SERVE   **GOOD SOURCE OF RESISTANT STARCH**

UNITS PER SERVE BREADS AND CEREALS **1** PROTEIN **0** FRUIT **1** VEGETABLES **0** DAIRY **0**   FATS AND OILS **0**

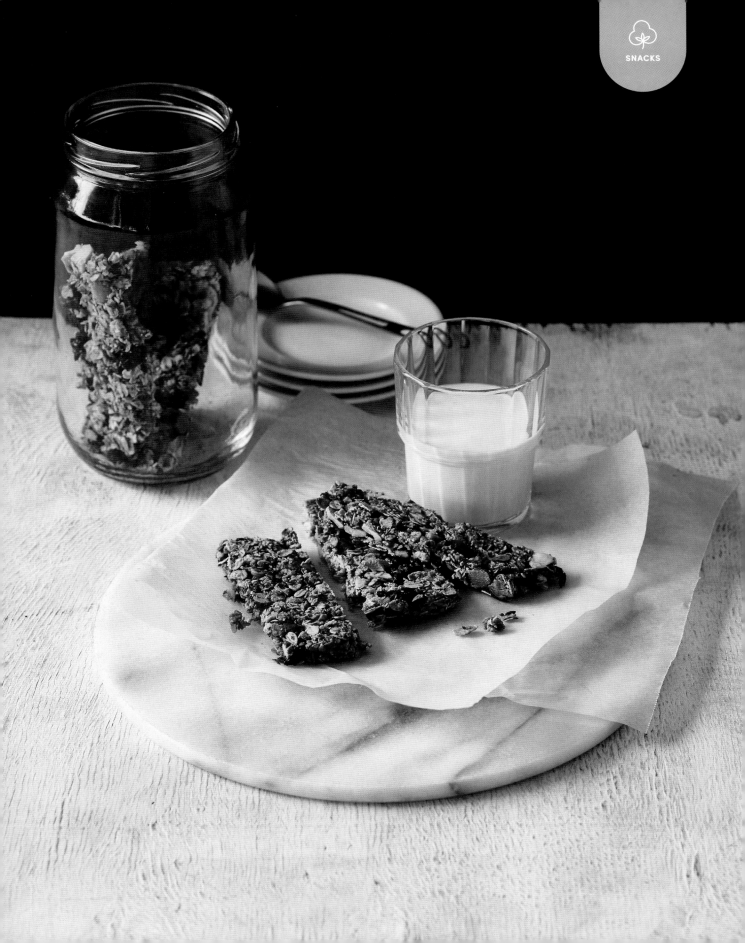

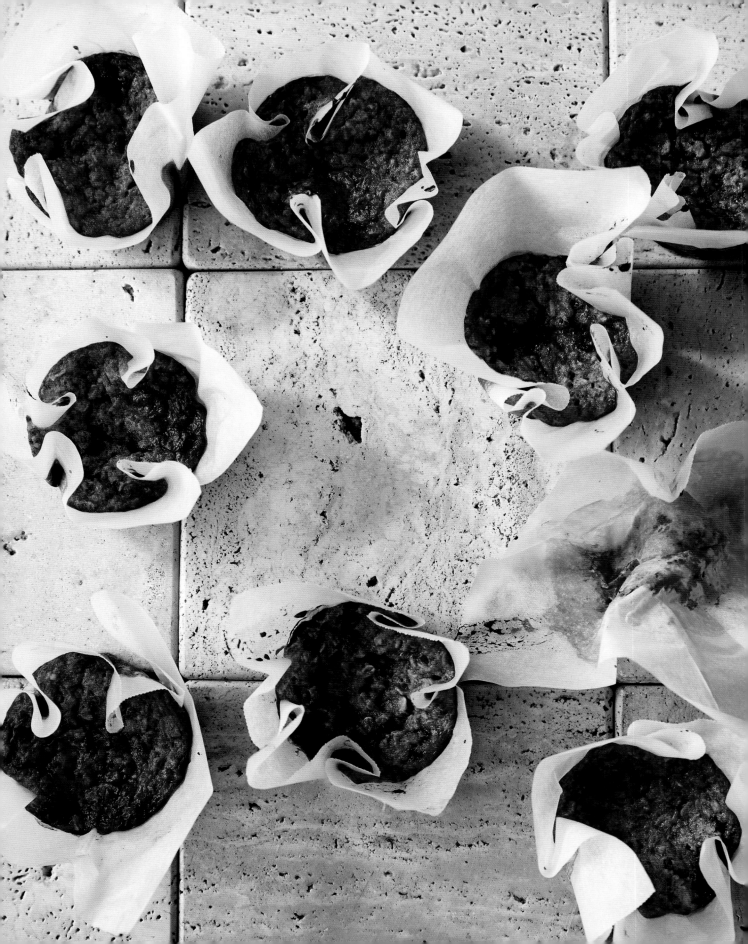

Banana *and* blueberry oat muffins

MAKES 12
PREPARATION 10 minutes
COOKING 15 minutes

100 g lactose-free natural yoghurt
⅔ cup (60 g) raw (natural) rolled oats
2 bananas, mashed
2 large eggs
1½ teaspoons baking powder
½ teaspoon bicarbonate of soda
finely grated zest of 1 small orange
125 g punnet fresh blueberries

Preheat the oven to 200°C (180°C fan-forced). Line a 12-hole muffin tin with paper cases.

Place the yoghurt, oats, banana, eggs, baking powder, bicarbonate of soda and orange zest in a food processor and pulse to just blend. Do not over-process; the mixture should still be fairly coarse. Fold in the blueberries.

Spoon the batter evenly into the paper cases, then bake for 15 minutes or until golden and a skewer inserted in the centre of a muffin comes out clean. Leave to cool in the tin for 5 minutes, then transfer to a wire rack to cool completely. Serve.

The muffins can be stored in an airtight container for up to 4 days or wrapped individually in plastic film and frozen for up to 1 month.

2 G FIBRE PER SERVE   **GOOD SOURCE OF RESISTANT STARCH**

UNITS PER SERVE BREADS AND CEREALS **1** PROTEIN **0** FRUIT **0.5** VEGETABLES **0**  DAIRY **0.5** FATS AND OILS **0**

Ricotta, pea *and* sweet potato mini frittatas

SERVES 4
PREPARATION 15 minutes
COOKING 20 minutes, plus sweet potato cooking time

olive oil spray, for greasing
100 g sweet potato, cut into
    5 cm × 2 cm strips, steamed and
    chilled overnight (see page 41)
½ cup (55 g) frozen peas
100 g reduced-fat ricotta, crumbled
⅔ cup (50 g) finely grated
    parmesan, plus 2 tablespoons
    extra for sprinkling
5 eggs, lightly beaten

Preheat the oven to 180°C (160°C fan-forced). Line a 12-hole muffin tin with paper cases and spray with olive oil.

Cut the sweet potato into 5 mm dice, then place in a bowl.

Cook the peas in a saucepan of simmering water for 3 minutes or until tender, then drain and run under cold water to cool. Add to the bowl with the sweet potato. Add the ricotta, parmesan, egg and freshly ground black pepper to taste, then stir to combine well.

Spoon the mixture evenly into the paper cases, then sprinkle with the extra parmesan.

Bake for 12–15 minutes or until the frittatas are light golden and set. Serve 3 per person, warm, at room temperature or chilled.

Use fresh ricotta from the deli for these frittatas. The ricotta sold in tubs at supermarkets has a different consistency.

2 G FIBRE PER SERVE   **GOOD SOURCE OF RESISTANT STARCH**

UNITS PER SERVE  BREADS AND CEREALS **0.5** ❋ PROTEIN **0.5** ❋ FRUIT **0** ❋ VEGETABLES **0** ❋ DAIRY **1** ❋ FATS AND OILS **0**

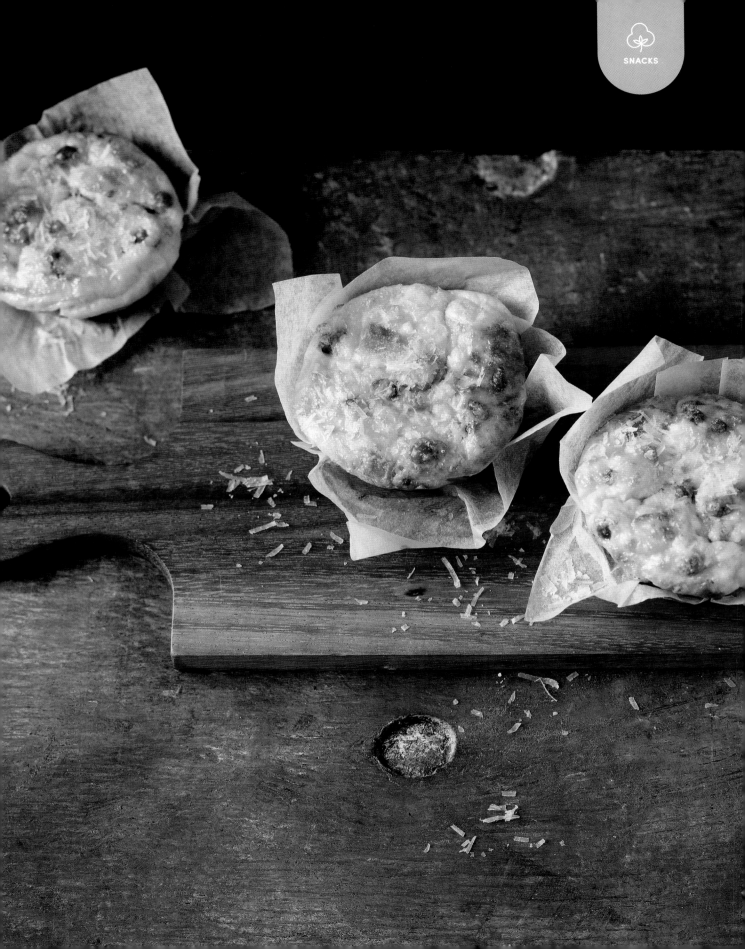

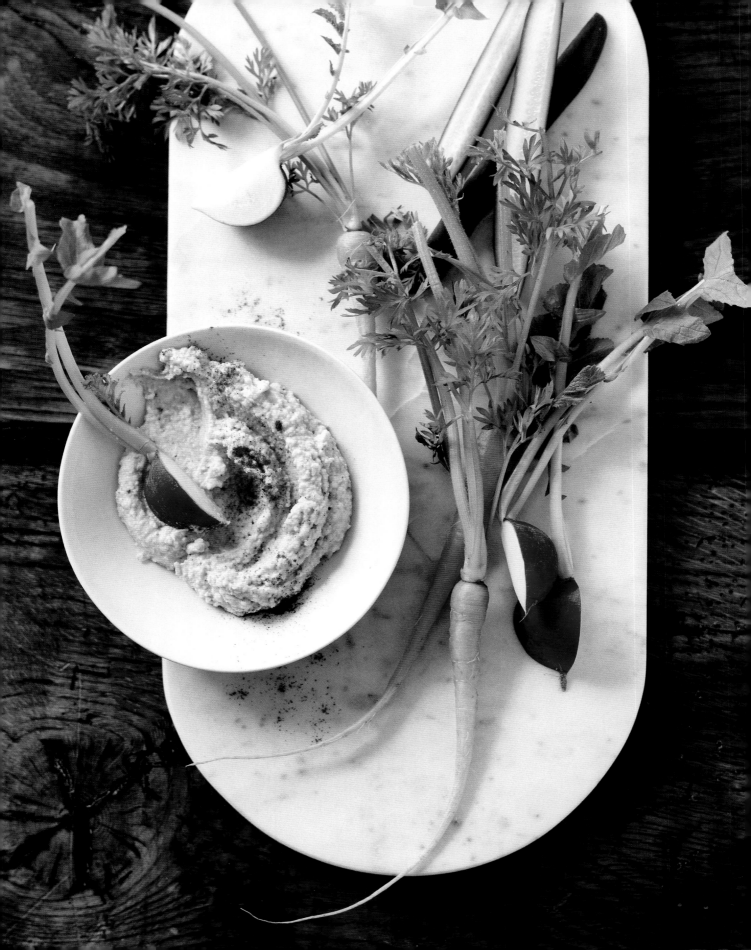

Roasted cauliflower hummus

SERVES 4
PREPARATION 20 minutes
COOKING 30 minutes

½ small or ¼ large head cauliflower, trimmed and cut into florets
1 large clove garlic
olive oil spray, for cooking
1 × 400 g tin salt-reduced chickpeas, drained, reserving the liquid, and rinsed
1 tablespoon tahini
juice of ½ lemon, or to taste
1 tablespoon extra virgin olive oil
sweet paprika, for sprinkling
1 bunch baby carrots, trimmed and well scrubbed
8 radishes, trimmed and halved
1 Lebanese cucumber, halved lengthways and cut into batons

Preheat the oven to 200°C (180°C fan-forced) and line a baking tray with baking paper.

Place the cauliflower and garlic on the lined tray in a single layer and spray with olive oil. Roast the cauliflower and garlic, turning occasionally, for 25–30 minutes until golden brown. Leave to cool, then peel the garlic.

Place the chickpeas in a food processor and add ¼ cup (60 ml) of the reserved chickpea liquid, then process until a very smooth puree forms. Add the cauliflower and garlic and pulse until well combined, then, with the motor running, add the tahini, lemon juice and olive oil and process until combined and very smooth; add a little more of the reserved chickpea liquid if a thinner consistency is preferred. Season to taste with freshly ground black pepper.

Transfer the hummus to a bowl, sprinkle with paprika and serve with the vegetables for dipping.

Enjoy this flavour-packed hummus with wholemeal Lebanese or pita bread cut into triangles (this will add 1 unit of breads and cereals per serve).

6 G FIBRE PER SERVE   **GOOD SOURCE OF RESISTANT STARCH**

UNITS PER SERVE   ❋   BREADS AND CEREALS **1**   ❋   PROTEIN **0**   ❋   FRUIT **0**   ❋   VEGETABLES **2.5**   ❋   DAIRY **1**   ❋   FATS AND OILS **2**

Spice-roasted chickpea *and* pea 'popcorn'

SERVES 4
PREPARATION 10 minutes
COOKING 40 minutes

2 cups (240 g) frozen peas, thawed
¼ teaspoon smoked paprika
1 teaspoon extra virgin olive oil

SPICE-ROASTED CHICKPEAS
1 × 400 g tin salt-reduced chickpeas,
    drained, rinsed and patted dry
½ teaspoon ground cumin
¼ teaspoon sumac
olive oil spray, for cooking

Preheat the oven to 190°C (170°C fan-forced). Line 2 baking trays with baking paper.

To make the spiced chickpeas, place the chickpeas in a bowl. Combine the cumin and sumac in a small bowl, then add to the chickpeas and toss to coat. Spread evenly over a lined tray in a single layer and spray with olive oil, then roast, stirring occasionally, for 35–40 minutes or until golden brown and crisp.

Meanwhile, gently pat the thawed peas dry with paper towel and place in a bowl, then add the paprika and olive oil and stir to coat. Gently spread out on the second lined tray, then add to the oven with the chickpeas. Roast for 30 minutes or until crisp, stirring them occasionally.

Leave the chickpeas and peas to cool on the trays, then store in separate airtight containers for up to 3 days.

7 G FIBRE PER SERVE   **GOOD SOURCE OF RESISTANT STARCH**

UNITS PER SERVE ❋ BREADS AND CEREALS **1** ❋ PROTEIN **0** ❋ FRUIT **0** ❋ VEGETABLES **0.5** ❋ DAIRY **1** ❋ FATS AND OILS **0**

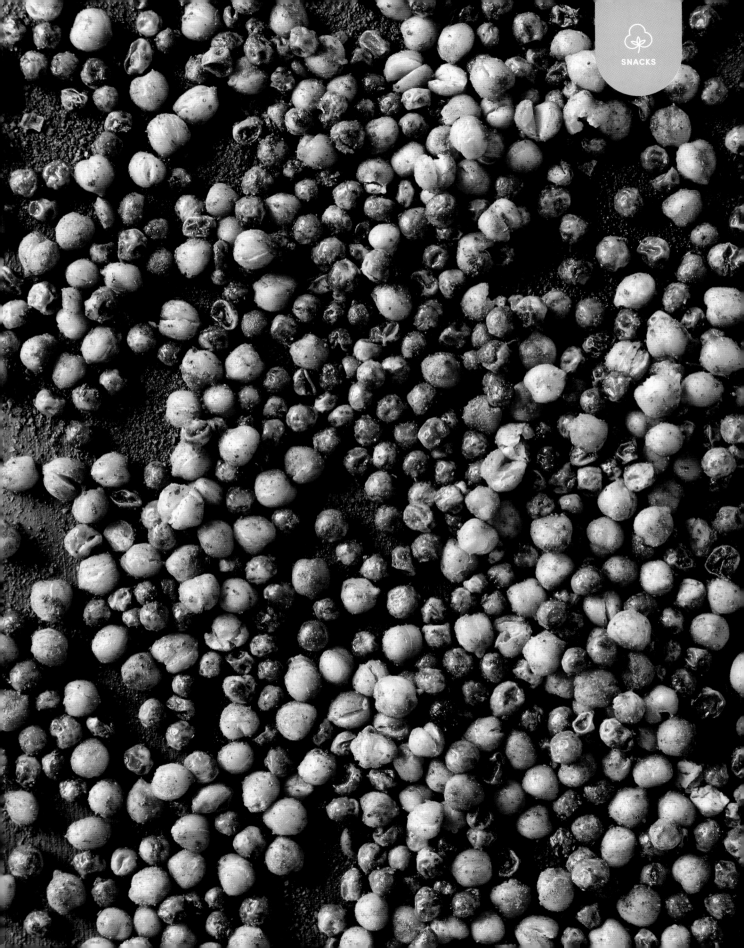

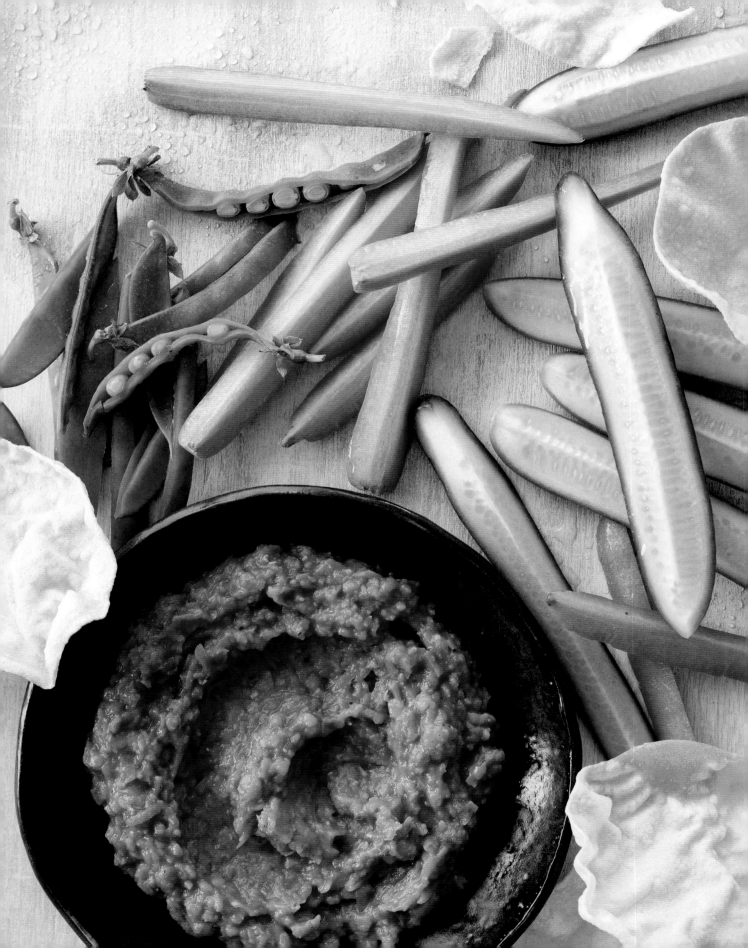

Dhal *with* pappadams

SERVES 4
PREPARATION 15 minutes
COOKING 30 minutes

100 g packet lentil pappadams
1 large carrot, cut into batons
2 Lebanese cucumbers, cut into batons
100 g snow peas, trimmed

DHAL

1 teaspoon garlic-infused olive oil
2 sticks celery, finely chopped
1 fresh long red chilli, seeded and
    finely chopped
1 cm piece ginger, finely grated
1½ teaspoons ground cumin
1½ teaspoons ground coriander
¾ teaspoon ground turmeric
½ teaspoon garam masala
1¼ cups (250 g) red lentils
½ cup (125 ml) salt-reduced
    tomato passata
1 carrot, coarsely grated

To make the dhal, heat a deep heavy-based frying pan with a lid over medium heat and add the olive oil. Add the celery, reduce the heat to low–medium, then cook for 3 minutes or until softened; add 1 tablespoon water, if necessary, to prevent the celery from sticking. Add the chilli and ginger and stir to combine, then cook for 30 seconds or until fragrant.

Add the cumin, coriander, turmeric and garam masala and stir for 30 seconds or until fragrant, then stir in the lentils, passata, grated carrot and 3 cups (750 ml) water. Increase the heat to medium–high and bring to a simmer, then reduce the heat to low and simmer, covered, for 20–25 minutes until the lentils are tender and thickened; add a little extra water if a thinner consistency is desired.

Heat the pappadams in the microwave according to the packet instructions.

Serve the dhal with the pappadams, carrot, cucumber and snow peas, for dipping.

14 G FIBRE PER SERVE   **GOOD SOURCE OF RESISTANT STARCH**

UNITS PER SERVE BREADS AND CEREALS **0.5** ✻ PROTEIN **0** ✻ FRUIT **0** ✻ VEGETABLES **2** ✻ DAIRY **0** ✻ FATS AND OILS **0**

Sweet potato oven fries

SERVES 4
PREPARATION 5 minutes
COOKING 50 minutes

1 sweet potato (about 600 g), cut into
    5 cm × 1 cm × 1 cm strips, steamed
    and chilled overnight (see page 41)
olive oil spray, for cooking

Preheat the oven to 190°C (170°C fan-forced).

Place the sweet potato in a roasting tin in a single layer, spray with olive oil and bake for 45–50 minutes or until golden and tender, turning halfway through the cooking time. Season with freshly ground black pepper and serve.

3 G FIBRE PER SERVE　　**GOOD SOURCE OF RESISTANT STARCH**

UNITS PER SERVE　✺　BREADS AND CEREALS **1**　✺　PROTEIN **0**　✺　FRUIT **0**　✺　VEGETABLES **0**　✺　DAIRY **0**　✺　FATS AND OILS **0**

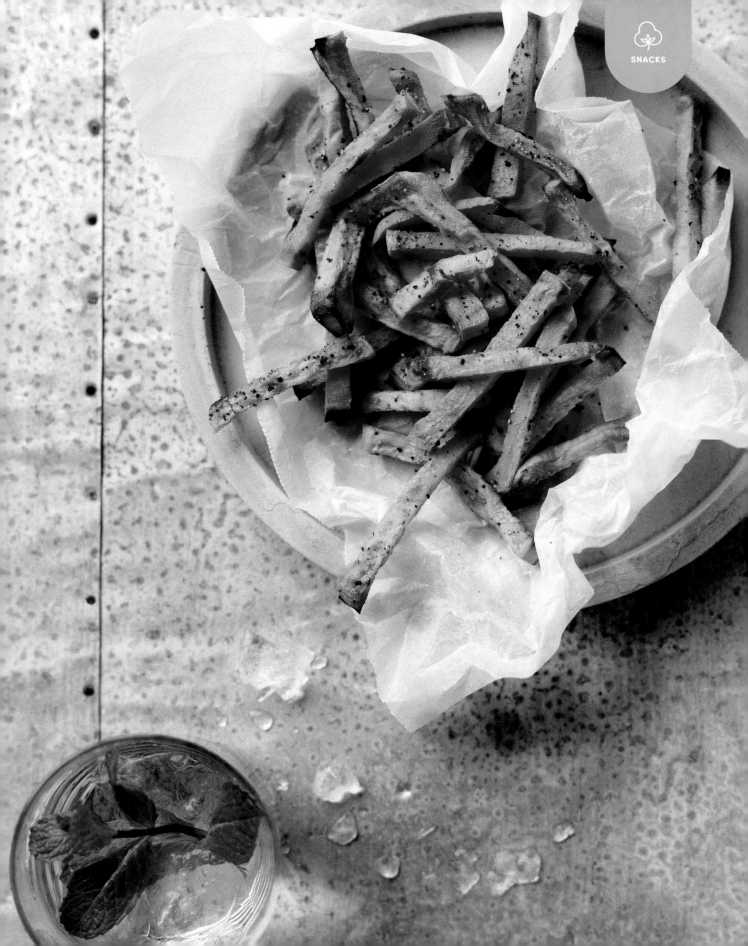

Zucchini roll-ups

SERVES 4
PREPARATION 20 minutes
COOKING Nil

2 zucchini, peeled into long thin ribbons
100 g salt-reduced Danish feta, crumbled
⅓ cup coriander leaves

CHILLI DRESSING

1 fresh long red chilli, seeded and finely chopped
1 tablespoon sesame seeds, toasted
¼ cup (60 ml) apple cider vinegar

To make the chilli dressing, mix together all the ingredients in a small serving bowl.

Lay the zucchini ribbons out flat on a work surface and top each with a little feta at one end, making sure you press down firmly to hold it in place. Top with a couple of coriander leaves, then roll up tightly to form a round resembling sushi.

Serve immediately with the chilli dressing for dipping.

2 G FIBRE PER SERVE | **LOW FODMAP**

UNITS PER SERVE ❋ BREADS AND CEREALS **0** ❋ PROTEIN **0** ❋ FRUIT **0** ❋ VEGETABLES **0.5** ❋ DAIRY **1** ❋ FATS AND OILS **0.25**

Italian corn thins

SERVES 4
PREPARATION 10 minutes
COOKING Nil

4 corn thins (thin cakes)
1 large tomato, thinly sliced into rounds
1 Lebanese cucumber, peeled into long thin ribbons
2 teaspoons red wine vinegar
½ cup small basil leaves
50 g parmesan, thinly shaved

Place the corn thins on a serving platter. Top with the tomato and cucumber and season to taste with freshly ground black pepper. Sprinkle with vinegar, then finish with basil leaves and shaved parmesan. Serve immediately.

2 G FIBRE PER SERVE | **LOW FODMAP**

UNITS PER SERVE ❋ BREADS AND CEREALS **0.25** ❋ PROTEIN **0** ❋ FRUIT **0** ❋ VEGETABLES **0.5** ❋ DAIRY **0.5** ❋ FATS AND OILS **0**

Lemony nuts *and* olives

SERVES 4
PREPARATION 10 minutes, plus standing time
COOKING Nil

10 natural almonds, finely chopped
1 stick celery, very thinly sliced
100 g pitted Sicilian green olives, halved
2 tablespoons lemon juice
1 tablespoon small rosemary leaves
    or ½ teaspoon dried rosemary
2 teaspoons garlic-infused olive oil

Place all the ingredients in a bowl and mix together well. Set aside for 10 minutes to infuse, then serve.

2 G FIBRE PER SERVE   **LOW FODMAP**

UNITS PER SERVE ❊ BREADS AND CEREALS **0** ❊ PROTEIN **0** ❊ FRUIT **0** ❊ VEGETABLES **0** ❊ DAIRY **0** ❊ FATS AND OILS **2**

Appendix

The **Bristol Stool Chart** is a visual diagnostic tool that classifies stools into seven categories. Consult your doctor if you notice any changes in your bowel habits, or you have any of the other symptoms outlined on page 27.

		BRISTOL STOOL CHART	
	Type 1	Separate hard lumps	SEVERE CONSTIPATION
	Type 2	Lumpy and sausage like	MILD CONSTIPATION
	Type 3	A sausage shape with cracks in the surface	NORMAL
	Type 4	Like a smooth, soft sausage or snake	NORMAL
	Type 5	Soft blobs with clear-cut edges	LACKING FIBRE
	Type 6	Mushy consistency with ragged edges	MILD DIARRHOEA
	Type 7	Liquid consistency with no solid pieces	SEVERE DIARRHOEA

Acknowledgements

A heartfelt thank you to Dr David Topping and Dr Trevor Lockett for their efforts in conceiving of this book and making it a reality.

We thank Associate Professor Peter Bampton, Gastroenterology Services, SA Group of Specialists; Professor Gordon Howarth, Gastroenterology Department, Women's and Children's Hospital; Nick Wray, Senior Gastro Dietitian and Co-Director of 360-me; and the following individuals from CSIRO Health and Biosecurity for providing their professional expertise in reviewing and advising on the book content: Dr Rob Grenfell, Director, Health and Biosecurity; Professor Manny Noakes; Professor Grant Brinkworth; Dr Nathan O'Callaghan, Dr Natalie Luscombe-Marsh and Dr Malcolm Riley. We would like to thank the many science leaders and co-investigators of our research exploring the area of diet and gut health for their contributions over several decades, and also thank the numerous individuals within the CSIRO teams that have conducted the research that underpin some of the important learnings articulated in this book, in particular the gut health, food analysis and clinical research teams.

Thank you also to the amazingly enthusiastic publishing and editing team at Pan Macmillan Australia – Ingrid Ohlsson, Virginia Birch, Megan Pigott, Naomi Van Groll, Nicola Young and Miriam Cannell – for your enthusiasm, insights and tireless support of this book, and your ability to bring science to the community. Thanks also to Kathleen Gandy and Tracey Pattison for the development and testing of the recipes; Sarah Odgers for her wonderful design; and the shoot team of Rob Palmer, Michelle Noerianto and Peta Dent for the beautiful photography.

Finally, thank you to the research volunteers for their ongoing participation in countless research trials that allow us to understand and learn about the factors that impact on gut health. It is due to our volunteers that we can make advancements in science.

Index

First published 2018 in Macmillan
by Pan Macmillan Australia Pty Limited
1 Market Street, Sydney, New South Wales
Australia 2000

A CIP catalogue record for this book is available
from the National Library of Australia:
http://catalogue.nla.gov.au

Design by Sarah Odgers
Photography by Rob Palmer
Prop and food styling by Michelle Noerianto
Recipe development by Kathleen Gandy and
    Tracey Pattison
Food preparation by Peta Dent
Editing by Nicola Young, Miriam Cannell
    and Rachel Carter
Colour + reproduction by Splitting Image
    Colour Studio
Printed in China by 1010 Printing International Limited

10 9 8 7 6 5 4 3 2 1